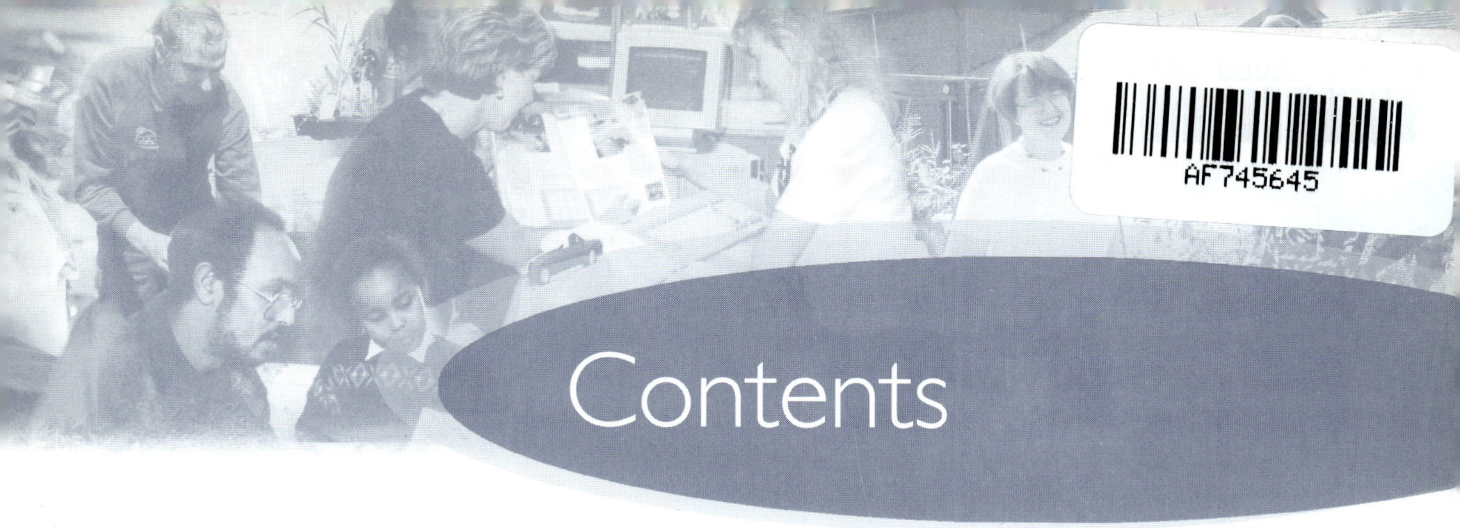

AF745645

Contents

LIBRARY
CHARLES FREARS CAMPUS
DE MONTFORT UNIVERSITY

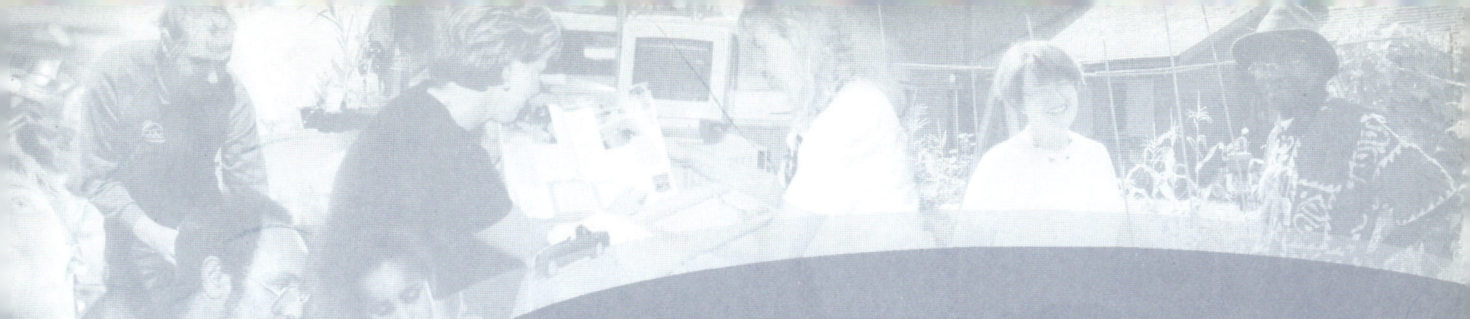

Introduction:
HOW TO USE THIS RESOURCE

This publication has been written to help the users and staff of mental health services think about citizenship and social inclusion. It is also written for people who live and work in other areas of the community and share our concern to ensure that people with mental health difficulties get a fair deal.

As a starting point

Each section discusses an aspect of social inclusion and citizenship and its relationship to mental health and comprises an introduction and a number of articles. The processes of social inclusion are complex and relatively untried. There is to date no list of simple instructions on how to 'do' it. However, this publication provides many starting points for discussion and action.

Although the contributions are arranged in a logical order, there are many relationships between the different sections. For example, the topic of mental health promotion is discussed in ***Section Two***, but also appears in ***Section Three*** and ***Four***. It is the nature of social inclusion that issues cannot be easily compartmentalised.

Responding to issues raised

Individual articles can be circulated to interested people for consideration. Key points for consideration appear at the end of each article. You may wish to bring together a group of people in your locality to discuss your responses to the issues raised.

The language of mental health

Words matter. Traditionally, those in power have used that power to define and name the experiences of others with words such as patients, psychiatric illness, acute treatment and rehabilitation. More recently, some individuals have reclaimed the territory with the

 © THE SAINSBURY CENTRE FOR MENTAL HEALTH, 2002

ordinary language of distress, crisis, survival, recovery and pride. Many writers have contributed to this publication and in doing so have used a variety of different terms. Rather than try to create a superficial consistency, these different words have been left in the text. Everyone has tried to write respectfully.

The use of examples

When examples are given in a publication of this kind, it can be misleading. People might assume the example is the best that anyone can do. The examples used are, in fact, the most interesting that we could find, but there may well be a number of much better projects in your locality.

Some people may assume that the project example is a recipe for success and try to photocopy the detail onto their own environment. Others may be tempted to point to what they perceive are the shortcomings of these 'flagship' projects, and ignore any lessons that are to be learnt. We hope that readers will look beyond the detail to the ideas, values and the goals that these projects espouse.

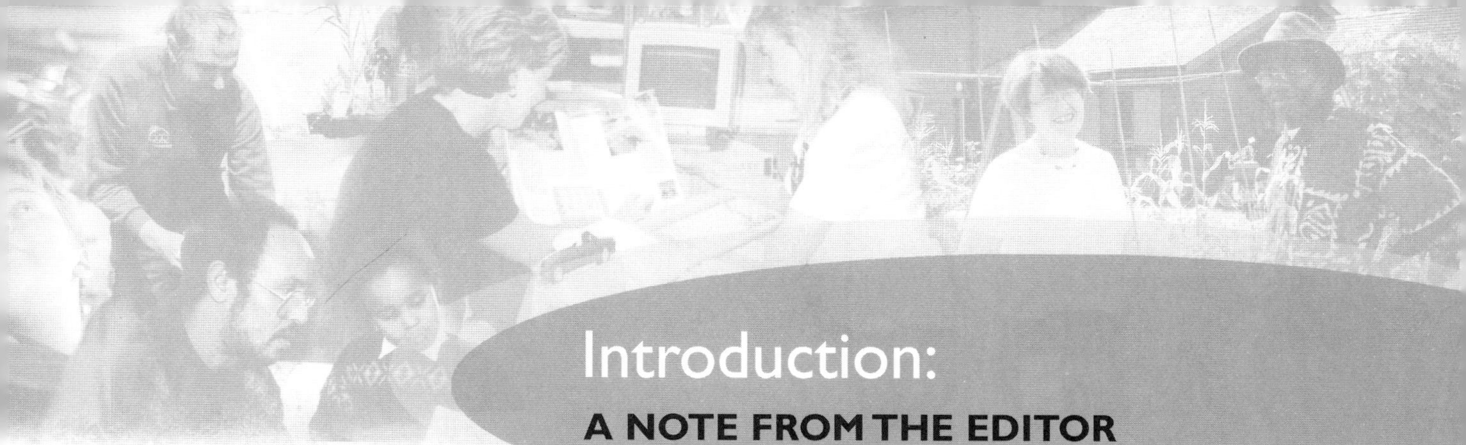

Introduction:

A NOTE FROM THE EDITOR

Peter Bates

One of New Labour's projects since coming into power has been the creation of a Social Exclusion Unit, responsible for tackling social exclusion across government departments. They have described social exclusion as

> "... *a shorthand label for what can happen when individuals or areas suffer from a combination of linked problems such as unemployment, poor skills, low incomes, poor housing, high crime environment, bad health and family breakdown.*"
> (Social Exclusion Unit, 1999)

A glance at the tabloid newspapers will show that this exploration is being undertaken in an environment that is often ambivalent and sometimes hostile. Media statements often emphasise the need to protect the community from people with mental health problems, promise zero tolerance towards homeless people, reinforce negative stereotypes of asylum seekers and make murderous threats against sex offenders.

The proposed revision of the *Mental Health Act 1983* strengthens powers to restrict the freedom of people with mental health problems who live in the community. In contrast, education, health and employment action zones, economic and community regeneration and a whole range of other government initiatives have been established with the explicit aim of combating social exclusion.

A wide range of evidence showing how people with experience of mental distress are subject to exclusion has been gathered over the past decade, culminating in the Mind Inquiry (Dunn, 1999). Some new local projects have sprung up in response to the focus on inclusion, while others have recognised that their longstanding programmes have been tackling social exclusion under other names.

Despite these initiatives, we have a sense that social inclusion and citizenship are either ignored or 'bolted on' to the existing mental health agenda. We wanted to look at the whole task of mental health services through the lens of inclusion. What issues would be raised? What would projects, care plans and performance indicators look like? The more work we gathered together, the more it became clear that social inclusion was not merely an attractive goal for mental health services – it was imperative.

A NOTE FROM THE EDITOR

Social inclusion is both new and old. It is as old as the effort to build a vibrant community, as old as the struggle to transform a stultifying bureaucracy, as old as the search for ways to harness each person's potential.

But there is new work to do. When friendships grow between mental health organisations and unlikely partners, such as museums, faith communities or business start-up agencies, all sorts of problems arise for which the policy handbook on the shelf has no ready-made answer. New work is needed to keep up with the aspirations of service users and creative staff who are eager to endorse and sponsor service users in voting, working and banking in the community.

This publication is not meant to be the last word in citizenship, social inclusion and mental health. The contributors have shared their perspectives and experiences on this emerging topic. In a year's time, some of them would want to write a very different article, as they grow in experience and plug some of the gaps in their personal understanding. We hope that it will stimulate a flurry of responses, inquiries, publications and most of all, improved practice.

Peter Bates
National Development Team

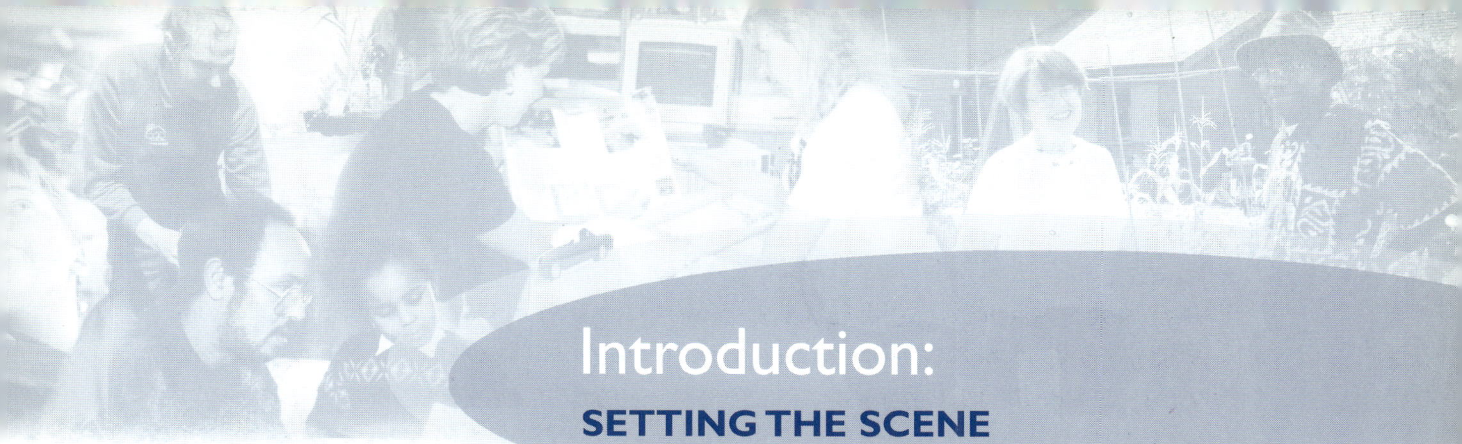

Introduction:
SETTING THE SCENE

David Morris

It is a great pleasure to introduce this resource on behalf of the Sainsbury Centre for Mental Health and six national partner agencies – Community Development Foundation, Disability Rights Commission, mentality, Mental Health Foundation, Mind, and the National Development Team.

This publication is one practical outcome of the Citizenship and Community Programme, a major national initiative on social inclusion, launched jointly by the Sainsbury Centre for Mental Health (SCMH) and Department of Health (DoH) in April 2001. Set in the context of new government policy on community regeneration and combating exclusion, the programme's aim is to bring together new and existing initiatives on inclusion. It aims to create, at policy, strategy and local practical level, the sustainable progress towards achieving social inclusion for citizens with mental health problems that the *National Service Framework (NSF) for Mental Health* (Department of Health, 1999b) requires.

Supported by some 30 partner organisations, this programme takes the interface between mental health services and community organisations as its starting point. It aims to: define citizenship and social inclusion in terms that will have practical implications for services and how they are provided; establish a collaborative process to building links between mental health services and mainstream community sectors; and develop and disseminate models of local community partnership which promote social inclusion.

The fact that we have been able to attract so readily the involvement of so many agencies and individuals to oversee and participate in this work, speaks volumes for the passion and urgency with which the objective of inclusive practice is being pursued. This is nowhere better represented than in this project, where six key organisations have joined with the SCMH to endorse the work of the many contributors who have enthusiastically committed their thoughts, skills and experience to this publication.

As the editor points out, we are not trying to present 'the last word' on inclusion, but to bring together some of the most interesting project examples and perspectives on theory that we have been able to find. We look at how the design and organisation of mental health services might be transformed to improve the ways in which they relate to the 'outside world'.

 © THE SAINSBURY CENTRE FOR MENTAL HEALTH, 2002

John Hutton, Minister of Health referred to this 'outside world' at the National Chief Officers' Mental Health Conference when he talked of needing to tackle *"the dead weight of bigotry and prejudice"* with which people who have severe mental health problems are so often confronted. Reducing stigma and discrimination; preventing the exclusion experienced by citizens with mental health problems must be an absolute priority for all services. Yet an active approach to inclusion which ensures real access to mainstream community opportunity, requires activity and engagement at the level of the individual and the local community.

How then is an active approach to inclusion to be pursued? As Peter Bates says in his introduction, we need to look at the whole task of mental health services through an 'inclusion lens'. Inclusion is not a 'bolt-on'. It is an essential ingredient in creating the fair access to services, decent standard of living and diverse relationships that we all aspire to.

The contributors to this resource book have been keen to replace the tired definition of community as the setting for services not provided within hospital, with others which suggest its capacity to support the recovery process. It is time to reframe our thinking on the value of communities.

We have a wide range of well-resourced government policies on community regeneration and renewal and it is now time to reorganise the mental health system around the possibilities so created. Thinking positively about the capacity of communities (whether neighbourhood, arts, faith, sports, employment or education based), to welcome people with mental health problems is an important step in restoring citizen rights lost through the impact of exclusion.

This publication illuminates this thinking and exposes us to new ideas of what might be possible, once we see communities and service users as reciprocally linked rather than automatically opposed through fear and prejudice.

We are offered some excellent examples of ways in which the ideas can be turned into practice, from the reasonable aspirations of people with mental health problems to their achievement in the ordinary social networks of which we are all a part.

Government policy on mental health has emphasised safety and support. The NSF for mental health specifies the essential service elements by which the policy objectives of safety and security) should be assured. However, the development of effective **support** systems in an era of standardised, targeted services provided by functionally specialist teams (such as assertive community treatment or crisis response teams) means we must find ways of re-engaging excluded service users with the wider, mainstream communities in which we all live, work, play and socially connect.

 © THE SAINSBURY CENTRE FOR MENTAL HEALTH, 2002

This is the real modernisation agenda in mental health and it is one to which the authors of this resource book have made a vital contribution. Their work as represented here is hugely appreciated. Thanks to the willingness of the many people to share their perspectives and experience, we have what we hope is a highly thought-provoking resource for others to build on.

If this publication even partially fulfils these objectives it will be due to the wisdom, drive and passion of its editor, Peter Bates, towards the principles and practice of social inclusion. You will see evidence throughout of Peter's vision and experience in this publication. It would not have been produced without his conceptual rigour and enviable ability to coax some very busy people to work within tight timescales.

I thank Peter for an enormous contribution both as contributor and as editor. I would like also to thank SCMH publications staff for all their help and advice, the partner agencies for extensive support and again, all the contributors.

In one sense, inclusion is simple. Citizens with mental health problems know it when they see, or, more correctly feel its impact. This is why the book says much, though perhaps not enough about the ways in which service users as direct experience trainers are the key resource in its achievement.

While the **experience** of inclusion lends itself to easy common sense definition, the process for its achievement does not, because it implies major cultural change, initially in health and social care organisations, but also beyond. This is a complex agenda in which policy and strategic support for localised good practice is as important as the practice itself. I hope that this resource book will have contributed to the discourse on inclusion at each of these three levels.

The views expressed by the contributors in this resource are their own. They are not necessarily those held by each of the partner organisations but we hope their inclusion encourages vigorous debate on this issue.

In the spirit of partnership and reciprocity, your responses, views and further contributions to the exciting change agenda that we have signalled here will, of course, be invaluable. Visit the discussion area of our website www.scmh.org.uk.

David Morris
Head of Citizenship and Community Programme
The Sainsbury Centre for Mental Health

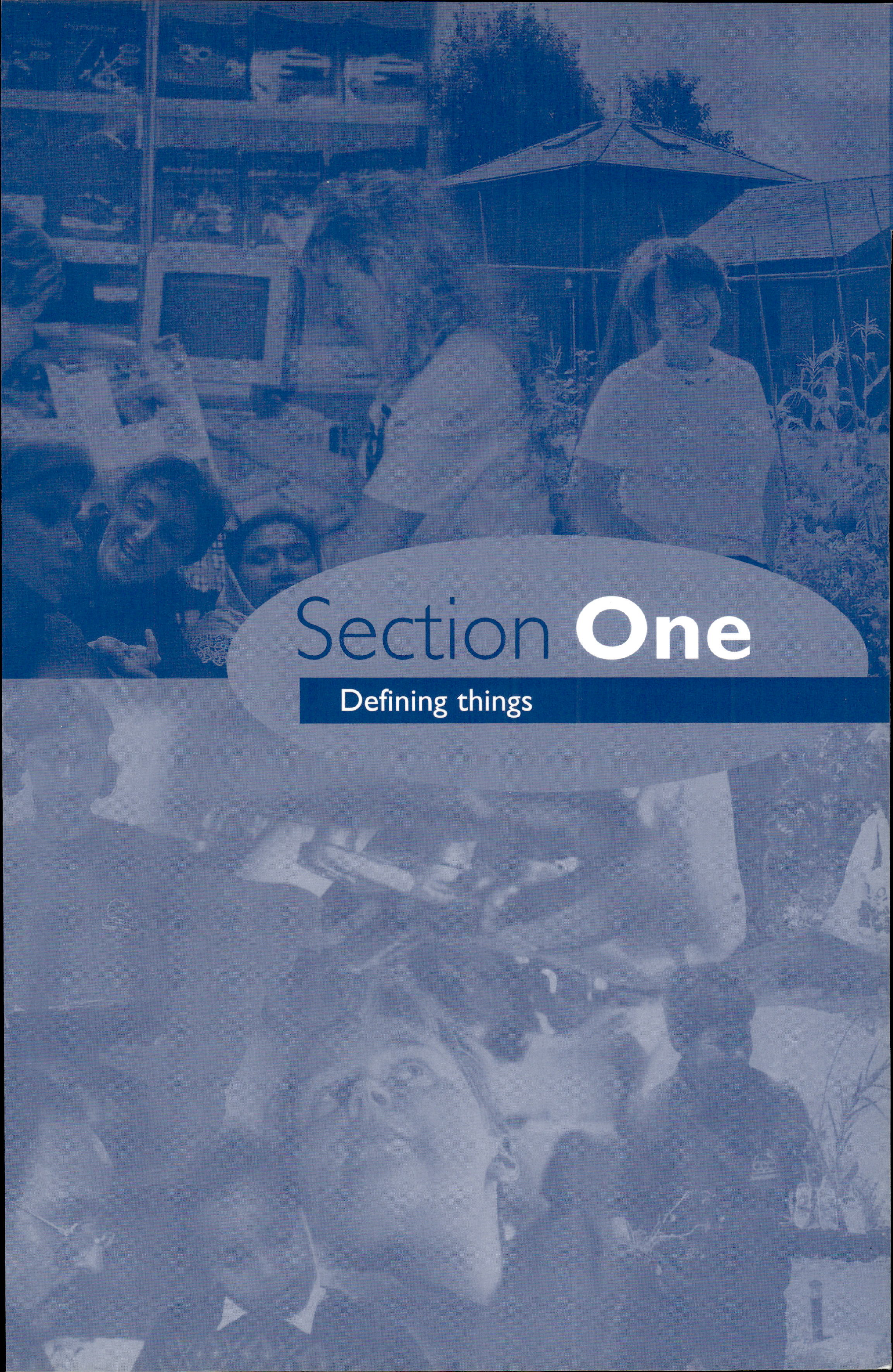

Section One

Defining things

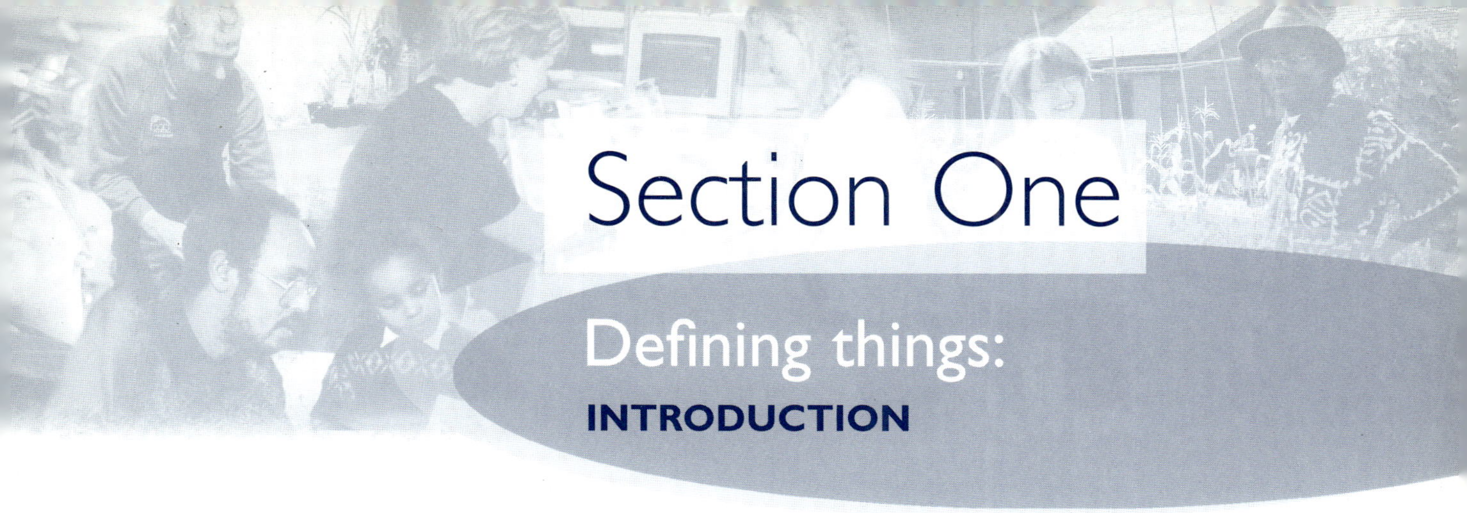

Section One

Defining things:

INTRODUCTION

Peter Bates

This section opens up some of the big ideas that underpin the book. Some readers will find much to stimulate discussion here, but others may wish to skip on to the more practical sections and return later.

Defining Inclusion offers one attempt to tease out some of the different perceptions that have informed practitioners and policy makers over recent years. Three definitions are presented – of inclusion as fair access to services and opportunities, inclusion as a decent standard of living and inclusion as an opportunity to enjoy a diverse range of relationships. All of these elements are shown to be essential to a comprehensive view of social inclusion and citizenship.

Many of the elements set out here impact on a whole range of people in society – not only those who are excluded through mental health difficulties, but also people excluded due to their ethnicity, gender, physical impairment or sexual orientation. Indeed, while it may be helpful to deconstruct the component parts of an inclusive lifestyle, there is also a need to analyse the multiple causes and processes of exclusion.

Distorted media representations combine with discrimination, hatred and structural injustices to form a complex web of interlocking forces that might exclude a mental health service user from a mainstream opportunity, then a black user from a white advocacy group, and then a blind person from a black majority organisation. Almost any list of 'devalued identities' could be slotted into the previous scenario to illustrate how this process of multiple exclusions can operate.

This publication does not have a separate section on specific multiple exclusions (such as the combined impact of mental health problems and ethnicity or mental health problems in combination with learning difficulty) or suggest many unique initiatives that promote inclusion for people in this situation. This is for three reasons:

- Most of the issues that are raised in the book are about everyone, rather than adopting a specific approach for any one group.
- We asked every contributor to address this issue in his or her article.

- We failed in our attempt to locate contributors willing to cover this topic from a solutions perspective rather than a diagnostic viewpoint. For a stimulating perspective on mental health and exclusion from the perspective of a black service user see Trivedi (forthcoming).

There is clearly room for additional work on this issue, and from time to time in this publication we will highlight areas that we believe need further investigation.

In *Defining Community*, Allyson McCollam and Julia White explore the variety of definitions of community that have emerged over the years. This discussion is important to prevent us from using the same words to talk about different things.

Whether people are developing active communities, providing care in the community, or engaged in community regeneration, a shared understanding of community is vital. One of the themes that is introduced here and recurs throughout the book is the tension between solidarity and diversity. Inclusion does not mean forcing people to fit into a static community, but rather the development of a dynamic, responsive community that is enriched by the participation of diverse peoples.

Allyson McCollam and Julia White then move on to present their work on *Defining Community Development*. Both the individual person and collective organisations share a joint responsibility for the well being of communities. Using community development approaches in mental health services is entirely legitimate and belongs alongside economic regeneration, environmental initiatives and democratic renewal.

Finally in this section, Fran Silvestri and Ken Jue from New Hampshire in the United States consider the role of *Inclusive Mental Health Services*. Fixing psychiatric symptoms is not enough, and an inclusive service will need to support individuals, families and whole communities to recover. We return to the theme of defining inclusive mental health services in the final section of this resource book.

© THE SAINSBURY CENTRE FOR MENTAL HEALTH, 2002

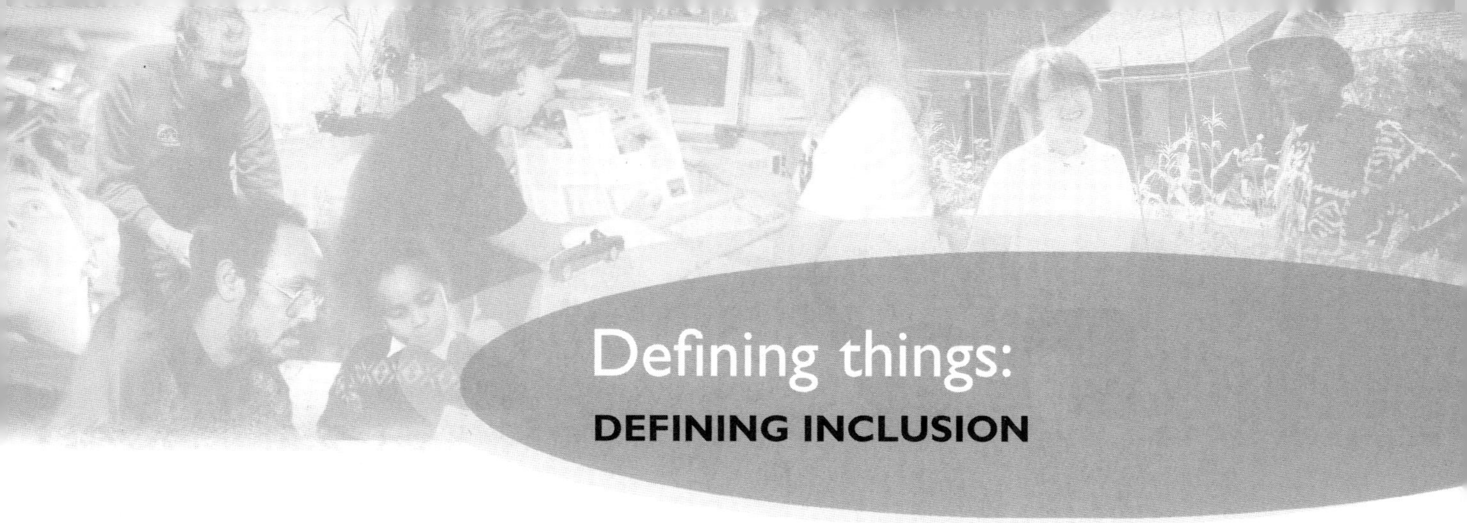

Defining things:
DEFINING INCLUSION

Peter Bates, Clive Miller and Paul Taylor

There are three ways in which mental health services vary in the extent to which they support social inclusion. These are summarised as access, standard of living and relationships. This article describes each of these in turn.

Inclusion as access

The first and simplest definition of social inclusion is to see inclusion as access. Within this frame of reference, an inclusive organisation is one that ensures all its activities serve the whole community. Hence inclusiveness applies not only to access to services and decision making around individual users but also to participation in planning and management and access to jobs.

Decision making about individual care and support is meant to fully involve service users but often falls short (Department of Health, 2000). Attempts to involve service users will only work if they are supported by empowerment. This involves empowering not only service users but also front line staff who play a critical role in decisions about the services that users receive.

Empowerment redefines the relationship between staff and service users, and staff and their managers as a partnership rather than patronage. Service users and front line staff are provided with information about the available services in languages and formats to suit a variety of communication requirements.

The Data Protection Act 1998 confirmed the right of service users to view information kept about them in most circumstances. Advocacy organisations are funded and welcomed when they support service users to understand information about the organisation and then the decision making process is amended to enable their considered responses to be taken seriously.

Access to services is often inequitable. This is especially the case for people from black and ethnic minority communities. Taking access seriously can lead to immediate results. For example, the over-representation of black and ethnic minority people within forensic psychiatry led to the provision of a counselling rather than drugs-based service to black service users in Birmingham which was met by an overwhelmingly positive response.

Service user knowledge and expertise is now recognised as a critical element in developing effective services and enshrined as 'consulting' within the Best Value framework for local authorities. If this resource is to be tapped, service users must be equal contributors in all the management, planning and quality assurance activities of the partner agencies. For example, enabling trained service users to carry out occasional 'access audits' by walking through the organisation's facilities and services and reporting to management on the barriers to full accessibility which they observe has enabled significant improvements to be made. In addition to this, there have been improvements in access to decision making by moving organisations away from secrecy towards transparency, as demonstrated by the impact of publishing the joint review inspections of social services departments.

Access is also about jobs. Since the workforce should be representative of the community it serves, the organisation should ensure that service users are represented on the staff team (Department of Health, 2000b).

Inclusion as a decent standard of living

The Social Exclusion Unit began with a broad remit which included paying some attention to communities of exclusion such as homeless people and pregnant teenagers (Cabinet Office, 1998), but it has lately focused most of its work on geographical exclusion – the so-called 'sink estates' (Cabinet Office, 2000).

However, there has been an increasing degree of clarity about the right of all citizens to be included in the good life that modern society has to offer. The Social Exclusion Unit focuses on four key areas of people's lives in which social exclusion is particularly prevalent and which have a pervasive impact on all other aspects of individual and collective well-being.

Everyone, including people who use mental health services, should be able to enjoy a good standard of health, develop their skills and abilities, earn a wage and live a life in the community in safety. Similarly, the *National Service Framework for Mental Health* Standard One (Department of Health, 1999b) demands that all people whose care is managed through the enhanced care programme approach should have a plan that addresses their needs for housing, employment and leisure.

Within this framework, an inclusive mental health service will address basic standard of living issues. Inclusive services will respond to psychiatric symptoms and offer treatment and a place of safety, but will also pay real attention to housing, education and employment. The community mental health team will include, or have direct access to: job coaching services, supported education and leisure, and a strategy that ensures high quality accommodation.

Information that is provided to service users will cover all these aspects of life rather than just health and social care services. At the heart of this work is a belief that people with mental health problems can make a practical and positive contribution to their communities as employees, neighbours and so on – and that these roles are a crucial element in recovery (Warner, 1985).

Inclusion as relationships

The reality for many people with mental health problems is that, apart from professionals and other service users, they have no other friends or community. This is why over the past 25 years an international network of people have been exploring strategies for creating a social mix between people who need support and other citizens (for mental health examples, see Carling, 1995; Sayce, 2000 and Wertheimer, 1997).

Whether working in schools, adult mental health or learning disability services, or as service users, relatives or advocates, this informal group shares a conviction that 'separate is not equal'. Within this framework, supported living replaces congregated staffed housing (Carling, 1995), real jobs replace day centres, and friendship with a diverse community of citizens (some of whom may have mental health problems) replaces comprehensive dependence on mental health staff and survivors.

An inclusive organisation that focuses upon relationships will push beyond the bald provision of a decent home and job to provide effective support for the development of good networks. Instead of 'whirlpool services' in which people find that increasing contact with psychiatric services means the systematic erosion of contact with informal networks, mental health teams will provide effective support to maintain these supportive and positive networks.

While friendships are magical and can never be artificially created, there are conditions that nurture friendship, such as respect and reciprocity (Home Office, 1999), and the inclusive organisation will be working with others for the development of a tolerant, welcoming community in which diversity is celebrated.

 © THE SAINSBURY CENTRE FOR MENTAL HEALTH, 2002

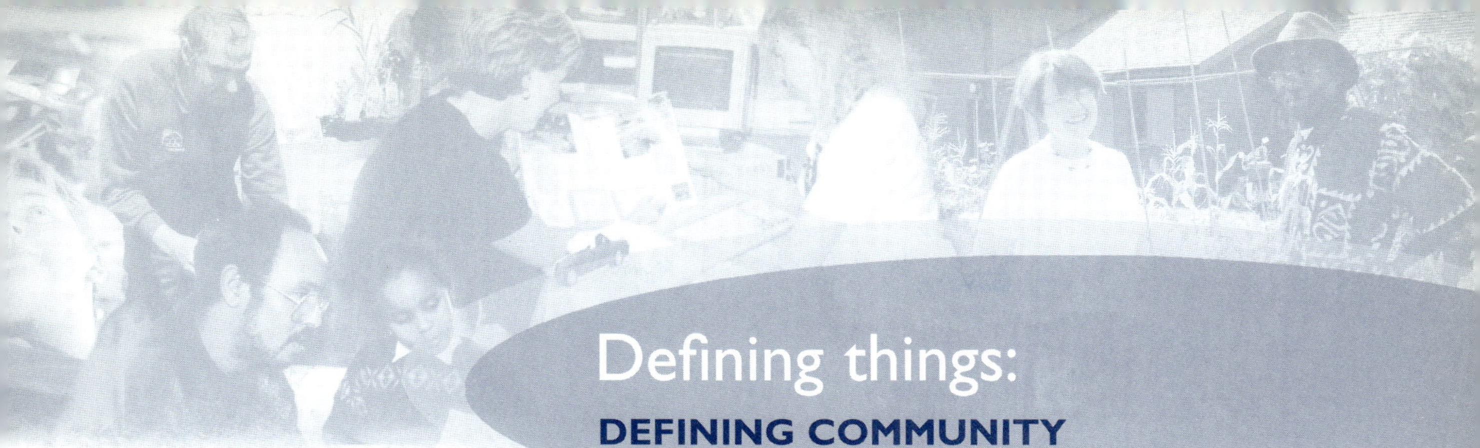

Defining things:
DEFINING COMMUNITY

Allyson McCollam and Julia White

Definitions of community

Definitions and understandings of community that derive from different theoretical and ideological models are likely to generate different accounts of the strategies and interventions that may be required to support and strengthen communities. This is not just an abstract theoretical issue, but also one that has a direct bearing on how we define the types of interventions required and the way that these are provided. Our constructions of community provide the rationale for our interventions and determine how we shape policy, strategy and action.

The following perspectives emerge from an overview of policy, research and practice discourse on community by the Scottish Development Centre for Mental Health (SDC, 2001a):

- Community can be seen as a useful vehicle to bring people together to tackle common problems and as a mediating structure between social institutions, large organisations/ bureaucracies and the individual. Communities can provide a forum and structure for people to engage with social policy and services that deliver policy objectives (Labonte, 1998).
- Much of the policy discourse on community is prescriptive in that it contains a vision of the community we should aspire to. For example, Scottish Office policy regards strong communities as a means of promoting social inclusion: strong communities are viewed as vital to an inclusive society and as a bulwark against the social exclusion of individuals and families (Scottish Office, 1999b).
- Definitions of community in the literature commonly make the distinction between communities based on the geographical areas or neighbourhood where people live and other communities, which centre on shared interests or identity (ethnicity, sexuality etc.).
- A further perspective on community has also been proposed, where a 'sense of community' denotes shared experiences and feelings, in addition to the social networks and patterns of behaviour that sustain them (Wilmott and Thomas, 1984).

 © THE SAINSBURY CENTRE FOR MENTAL HEALTH, 2002

In a study that explored theoretical and practice perspectives on community mental health and well-being, the following key issues were identified:

- The importance of how community identity is ascribed and by whom. Practitioners and community activists alike reported considerable discomfort and frustration in having to work with communities created ostensibly for administrative convenience or to deliver the latest set of policy objectives.
- By contrast practitioners and community activists considered that community was defined by the values that held them together and differentiated them from other communities (SDC, 2001a)

In the context of community development, it is important to consider what these differing perspectives on community imply about the role of community members, about the basis for community membership and how eligibility is determined.

- Choice versus ascribed belonging: people may decide to be part of a community. They may be told that they are part of a community, for example people with mental health problems are increasingly regarded as part of a wider disability movement, but may not perceive themselves as such.
- Being in a community versus being active in a community: people who live in an area do not necessarily wish to become active; whereas someone who joins a local environmental group may do so in order to campaign for change.

We should not be led into romanticising the notion of community, however, and need to be aware that communities can be closed as well as close (Forrest and Kearns, 1999). A distinguishing feature may be the extent to which communities can combine a capacity to maintain internal cohesion with a capacity to be outward looking and sustain links that reach outside.

 © THE SAINSBURY CENTRE FOR MENTAL HEALTH, 2002

Relationship between individual and community

An issue that is perhaps less well developed in the literature is the relationship between the individual and community, the extent to which this evolves over time and the factors that influence that relationship. A key aspect is the process of negotiation and accommodation the person uses to determine and adjust their relationships with their networks and ties. Those working in services need to be aware of their role in supporting, facilitating and sometimes mediating those relationships, and to be conscious that they can also undermine them, inadvertently or deliberately.

There are a number of factors that appear relevant here. Firstly, the individual's own internal resources can influence their responses to external events and to the support available. Secondly, a person's ability to engage with community may be influenced by their previous personal experiences of relationships and attachments in general and their perceptions of the benefits that may or may not be associated with community membership.
A third factor is the role that the individual can expect to play or wishes to play within a network of ties and relationships. Some interpretations of community contain connotations of mutuality, of an interaction that involves giving and receiving. Engagement with public services, including mental health services, tends to cast the individual as a beneficiary or recipient.

In addition, for the individual, developing connections and ties with others entails managing the tension between autonomy and independence. The balance between the rights and responsibilities of individuals and those of the community is a core issue in considering the meaning of community in relation to mental health.

There can be a tension between efforts to encourage participation on the one hand, and on the other pressures to require people to adhere to norms and expectations associated with the social group. It is important therefore to explore the meaning of solidarity and diversity and to consider possible differences in the meaning ascribed to ties and affiliations within and between different generations, genders and ethnic groups.

Without such an understanding, the goals of inclusion and normalisation can give an illusion of conformity, homogeneity and connection and only hide from view those who are 'non-members', whether through choice or through exclusion. The tension in practice between strong communities and social inclusion is amply illustrated by the all too familiar experience of many people with mental health problems who find that the communities they encounter are not tolerant or accepting.

 © THE SAINSBURY CENTRE FOR MENTAL HEALTH, 2002

Key points

- Each mental health project carries its own understanding of community– even if this is hidden. What do the publicity materials and practices of your organisation reveal about this?
- Who defined your community and set the boundaries of your work?
- How are service users supported in (a) choosing which communities to join and (b) achieving their preferred level of participation?
- Do you have a clear idea of the user's previous experiences of community membership and future ambitions as a community member?
- How have you tailored your work in response to differences between generations, genders and ethnic groups?

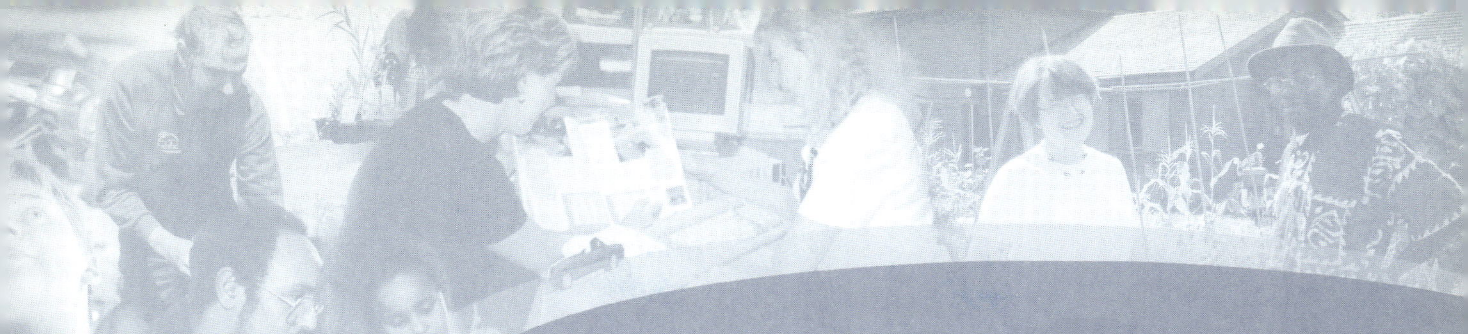

Defining things:
DEFINING COMMUNITY DEVELOPMENT

Allyson McCollam and Julia White

Introduction

This article explores the role of community development in promoting the mental health and well-being of individuals and communities. It begins with a brief consideration of the UK policy context and then moves on to examine the relevance of community development approaches in work that aims to promote mental health and well-being. It concludes by presenting the mandate for services to work in this way and identifies the challenges that implementation of these approaches bring for health and social services.

It draws on a range of material: government policy, policy analysis, social theory, and empirical research. It is also informed by the work of the Scottish Development Centre for Mental Health (SDC) in supporting policy and practice development in relation to the promotion of mental health and well-being and in facilitating debate and discussion in Scotland in this area.

Core themes

The discussion that follows is shaped around two core themes. Firstly, social support/social capital (see article by Sarah Hean in ***Section Five*** of this resource) are valuable resources that contribute to mental health and well-being. It is therefore important to look at what mental health services can do to encourage, develop and sustain these assets for the benefit of individuals, families and communities.

Secondly, mental health and well-being are affected by deep-seated structural/socio-economic factors. The experience of individuals and of communities is often one of disempowerment and an inability to influence or impact on those areas that most directly affect people's lives: housing, employment, income, and education.

Our proposition is therefore to explore what community development can offer on each of these fronts, both in building links and connections between people and in empowering and enabling people to have more influence and control.

The importance of community from a policy perspective

The concept of community figures prominently in discussions of health and well-being and of social justice in recent and current government policy. A close reading of such sources (e.g. Scottish Office, 1999a) indicates that health and well-being are regarded as both an individual and a social responsibility and imply that individuals have to take responsibility for themselves and for others. It follows from this analysis that the aspiration to promote social inclusion involves creating the conditions that foster the responsibility that individuals take for their own health and that of others.

At the same time, current UK health policy contains explicit recognition of the social and economic determinants of health and therefore of mental health. There is, for example, a commitment in the Scottish Social Justice Strategy to build strong, inclusive communities and to reduce inequalities between communities as well as to involve communities in renewal processes.

Policy that impacts on health and well-being therefore juxtaposes two distinct strands. The first stresses individual rights and responsibilities and looks to citizens to play their part more fully, collectively and individually in achieving improved health and well-being. The second acknowledges inequalities in health and its structural determinants, and recognises the need for multi-sectored approaches and longer-term vision to tackle such complex issues.

Why community development?

Community development approaches have a key role to play in promoting mental health and well-being. Indeed, it is possible to argue that community development is a necessary way of working to achieve the desired outcomes in mental health policy and social inclusion.

Why is it relevant to mental health?

- Community development is about working in partnership with individuals and established groups, to enable them to gain more control over their environment and over their lives.
- Empowerment can be seen as a means to improved well-being and as an indicator of better well-being. Labonte (1998) regards the sense of control over one's life as a feature of well-being.

 © THE SAINSBURY CENTRE FOR MENTAL HEALTH, 2002

- Community development can be a way for individuals and groups to negotiate their relationship with the outside world and with social institutions, including policy makers, planners and service providers.
- Community development builds bridges between people on the basis of their shared experiences and interests. It values that experience as a means of understanding the issues and developing strategies for change.

Community development is founded on the following values:

- A social model of health that recognises social and environmental influences of health and that values individual perception and experience of health.
- A focus on the collective as well as on the individual, to help reduce isolation and to develop mutual support and shared experiences of problems and solutions.
- Participation and democracy (Jones, 1999).

Key features

Community development aims to:

- enable people to make choices and decisions from a position of knowledge;
- support and develop individuals and groups to achieve individual and community empowerment;
- promote collective action and self-help;
- work to an agenda set by those who are involved, not one imposed by others;
- enable community members to participate in the process of identifying, exploring, understanding and addressing issues of concern;
- work through and build on existing networks and structures;
- target change and development in the social environment and social relations, including extending opportunities for participation and involvement.

Mandate for mental health services to use community development approaches

Health authorities are now required to articulate their vision and strategy to improve the mental health and well-being of the population they serve. This is in line with the World Health Organisation's Health 21 Strategies for Mental Health, which include the development of individual and community ability to recognise and deal with stress and its root causes.

 © THE SAINSBURY CENTRE FOR MENTAL HEALTH, 2002

Health 21 envisages that the main strategies for action will entail multi-sectored approaches to tackle health determinants and participatory health development processes involving relevant partners for health, including the local community.

This agenda has significant implications for mental health services in relation to:

- the priority that can/will be assigned to promotion and prevention;
- the roles and functions that statutory health and social services can play in this area of work, alongside the voluntary sector and other services such as employment and housing;
- the capacity and skills needed to promote mental health and well-being among communities;
- the nature of alliances and partnerships required with communities and with other agencies and services.

Community development is a potentially powerful resource that facilitates collaborative working across sectors and boundaries (statutory and voluntary, health and social services, professional and user). It can also be used in a variety of settings, such as schools, workplace or neighbourhood, and on different levels: with individuals, leading into collective work with established groups, within a service or organisation, or within a local network of organisations.

Challenges and possibilities

Community development approaches can pose challenges to those who work in mental health services in a number of ways:

- It is founded on a model of health that health professionals may be familiar with but may not have utilised as the basis for practice.
- It entails a fundamental reworking of the relationship between professionals and service users and sets high value on the experiences and understanding of the latter.
- Issues of power and power relationships have to be explicitly acknowledged and addressed.
- Empowerment and participation means that 'the system' is exposed to challenge and questioning, which generates expectations of change.
- This has wider implications for accountability and scrutiny if community members and those who use services are to have an active role in monitoring and evaluation.

© THE SAINSBURY CENTRE FOR MENTAL HEALTH, 2002

BOX 1 Eight ways to support community development

Health and social services can promote and support the use of community development approaches in many ways; both within mental health services and to promote the mental health and well-being of the populations they serve.

1. Structure organisations and deliver services in ways that foster supportive aspects of communities and do not undermine them through policies that weaken the capacity of communities.
2. Find more creative and imaginative ways for people to be heard.
3. Guard against the development of communities that lead to collective marginalisation/exclusion of certain groups of the population (ghettos are communities after all).
4. Use the wealth of experience that exists to develop a better understanding and appreciation of effective interventions and practice.
5. Take the longer-term perspective on change and development, ensuring that this is recognised in how such work is evaluated.
6. Be clear about the relationship between services for people with identified mental health needs and wider work focusing on mental health promotion. Without clarity about how these strands link, long-term users of mental health services will be concerned that they stand to lose out if resources are diverted into new work promoting mental health.
7. Ensure that performance management systems support community development and do not cut across it. Introduce targets and incentives to signal that this area of work is valued.
8. Be clear about the difference between working in a community and living in it. There are likely to be different perceptions of community depending on whether you are providing services or trying to use them.

Where do we go from here?

There is no denying that community remains a contested and difficult concept that should be handled cautiously, with due regard for the possible negative consequences of misapplication. For example, although the links between the environment and well-being and between social support and well-being are now generally recognised, it would be a mistake to view community as the sole source of health and well-being. This would only serve to shift the onus of responsibility for ill health away from individuals to communities (SDC, 2001b).

To take forward the promotion of mental health and well-being, we need to give further consideration to what community membership – belonging and connectedness – means for different people and how we can help to build that. We need also to understand better what it is that enables communities to be outward looking and have ties with the outside world, close but not closed.

Policy gives a clear mandate to use community development. It is important however, that those in positions of leadership in mental health take cognisance of what is required to support and sustain it and address the factors that impinge on capacity for community action and social change, which are both structural and cultural.

Community development offers a means of understanding and working with communities to bring about social change. The terrain of community development is well charted by some, but unknown to many others. At present, many of those with experience in community development remain on the fringes of mental health services. We need to find ways of legitimising this work and establishing stronger links with other parts of the local service system and at the same time respect and protect the participatory, inclusive ethos that characterises community development.

There are opportunities to promote mental health not just through health policy, but also through social justice and the pursuit of joined-up government. Indeed, one of the most striking developments in recent mental health policy in the UK is the message that the desired policy goals cannot be achieved by mental health services alone.

The aspiration to enhance the mental health and well-being of individuals and communities requires that we extend our thinking, planning and practice into wider expanses (Scottish Public Mental Health Alliance, forthcoming). We need to reconsider the way in which we understand and interpret community mental health if we are to generate effective solutions.

© THE SAINSBURY CENTRE FOR MENTAL HEALTH, 2002

Key points

- Individuals carry some degree of responsibility for their own health and the health of the community. How is this played out in local mental health services?
- How are you contributing to a multi-sector approach and long term vision that tackles the structural determinants of mental distress?
- Who is working on WHO Health 21 in your area and what are they doing?
- What resources and skills are needed to promote mental health in your community?
- Adopting a community development approach means that power shifts from professionals towards service users. How are the various interest groups being supported to make this shift?
- How do we support communities to be 'close but not closed'?

Acknowledgements

The authors would like to acknowledge the contribution of Professor Steve Platt, Director of the Research Unit in Health, Behaviour and Change, the University of Edinburgh, to the research project on 'Community Mental Health and Well-being' (SDC, 2001a) referenced in this article and in the previous article on *Defining Community*.

 © THE SAINSBURY CENTRE FOR MENTAL HEALTH, 2002

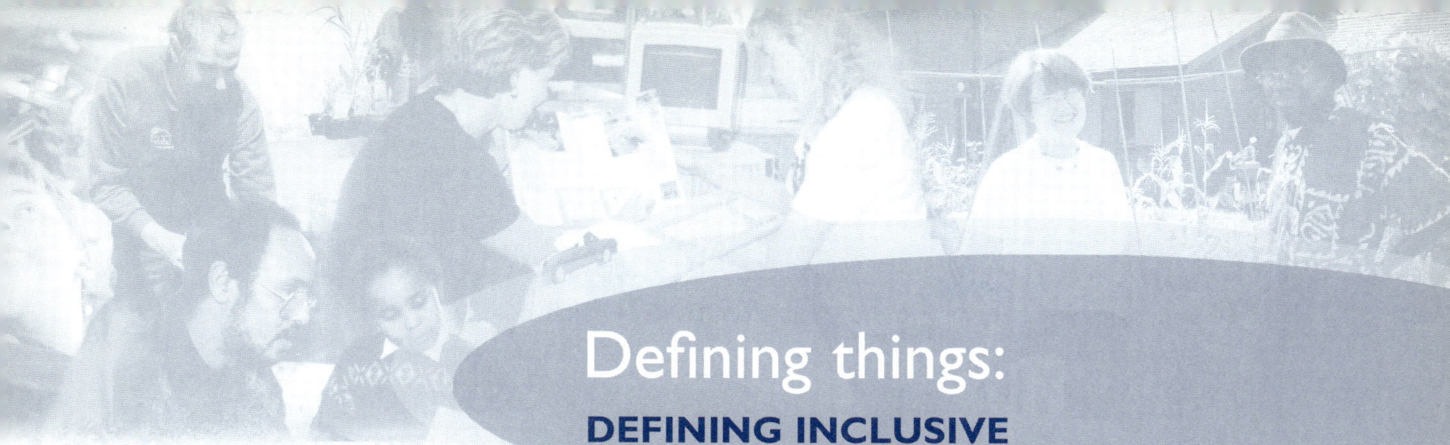

Defining things:

DEFINING INCLUSIVE MENTAL HEALTH SERVICES

Fran Silvestri and Ken Jue

In the 1950s an international movement began to decrease the number of people held in large psychiatric institutions. With the advances in medications and civil rights, the belief developed that people living in those institutions should be allowed to return to their communities and be cared for there. As a result community mental health centres began offering a variety of services to support those discharged from these institutions.

Throughout the past 40 years, governments and providers have launched a variety of services that were specialised and community related. These services have provided some lasting supports, but people have also complained about lack of access and meaningful work, poor housing, homelessness and poverty.

Three groups who often complain are families disappointed with mental health services, service users who feel the services are not effective, too controlling and do not respect them, and the media which expresses concern about safety.

There is an alternative. This is to return to the concept of community and a belief that providers must be family and service user focused, providing supports that are needed rather than moving service users through pre-arranged service systems. It will take time and effort to reform how we think of providing care, but if successful, the result will be lower cost and better outcomes for service users, their families and the community.

The responsibility for mental health care lies with the larger community in partnership with those who use mental health services and with their families and friends. The responsibility of a community mental health centre (CMHC) in the USA is to facilitate and promote the notion that the total community is the responsible party.

Providers of mental health services should support the community and service users and aim to link them with the community resources that can help them to achieve their goals. The CMHC supports the service user's ultimate inclusion in mainstream community life.

What providers have traditionally designed are services, rather than a comprehensive community support system that assists service users to achieve the outcomes that they want. We propose that the essential players in the support system include the service users,

 © THE SAINSBURY CENTRE FOR MENTAL HEALTH, 2002

their families and friends and the wider community (which includes at least the providers and commissioners of services). The way in which we should assist the support system is based on three key principles:

- a 'recovery' philosophy of care;
- integration;
- accountability (a system to assure effective and efficient use of resources).

Systems of care should focus on these three principles and aim to build the capacity within the community to support individual service user recovery. This is achieved through an aggressive individual service user focused recovery plan and the integration of relationships among service users, their families and the wider community.

Fundamental to the achievement of this capacity building is the establishment of a quality process that assures resources are utilised efficiently and are effective in assisting service users to achieve the quality of life that they seek.

The design of the mental health system would revolve around the development of capacity:

- Developing capacity in the general community requires a wider and more global effort to elicit change, i.e. targeted interventions to help the community recover from its stigmatisation and misconceptions about mental illness. Since influencing community perceptions takes a long time, gains in community capacity have to be measured over the long term.
- Designing interventions or supports for service users and families can be done more quickly and more directly with results seen in shorter periods of time.

Working on both levels is essential. For example, when a service user begins a job it is very useful to have the community (whether it is colleagues on the shop floor, a manager or personnel officer) understand about mental health care.

A recovery approach

People who use mental health services want to recover from their illness: they do not intend to become over-dependent. The mental health system must focus on assisting service users to recover and live independent and meaningful lives – which they define for themselves. The following summarises an approach based on our experiences in the Monadnock region of New Hampshire, USA.

© THE SAINSBURY CENTRE FOR MENTAL HEALTH, 2002

The individual

The primary objective of working with individuals is that they will be able to recover and thrive. Success depends upon a recovery-based approach in service delivery. There are many designs for a recovery-focused process within the care planning systems and models of assessments. We believe that any well designed step by step process can work, so long as certain principles are applied that are the foundations of a recovery-based care approach. The four fundamental principles are:

- focus on individual strength;
- acknowledgement and encouragement of individual responsibility;
- self determination;
- individual need for a life purpose and meaning.

To effectively work in a recovery-focused way, we need to believe in the individual's capacity to recover and thrive within the community. We believe emphasising individual strengths is more helpful than any combination of drugs and day programmes.

Part of this move toward recovery is the realisation that service users must be responsible for themselves. Service users are capable of determining what they want and can be held responsible for their care plan. Neither self-determination nor self-responsibility can occur without the other. It should be assumed that the recovery process is the responsibility of the individual, not the provider or commissioner. Individuals are responsible for themselves, no matter how ill they are.

When we try to establish what individual service user outcomes should be, we must not forget that a fundamental need for individuals is the search for life meaning, their purpose for living. Mental health is not just a physical health issue. It goes beyond the physiology of the brain. We must assist the individual to go beyond managing their symptoms. Many service users often speak about their sense of hope. This can translate into their desires, purpose and meaning for the future.

Recovery from any illness is achieved when the individual is included back into the community. This has been a fundamental principle within the community mental health movement. To achieve this the mental health system should help individuals participate in the general community in whatever roles they choose, as a political activist; a person with a social network of friends, families and peers; or with a home and a career.

To do this means going beyond simply referring individual service users to other mental health agencies and expands toward the notion of partnerships or collaboration, for example, with those who can provide housing and jobs.

 © THE SAINSBURY CENTRE FOR MENTAL HEALTH, 2002

If each community's mental health system is truly community-based then its actions can assist service users to move toward inclusion and links within the community. The community mental health centre itself has to be an example of this integration. It must be connected as a community contributor, be politically active and must understand how to create links to open living and career opportunities for those service users who use long term supports.

The family

Voluntary organisations have played a major role in helping families to deal with the effect of having a family member with a mental health problem. When the services are poor and ineffective, families suffer tremendously. The system of care has to pay attention to these needs. Families also need to go through their own recovery process. We can assist families in building their capacity to cope with their experiences and offer guidance on what they can do to assure that their communities respond positively.

Recovery for family members is built on three major facets: their responsibility to support their family member, to be politically active to ensure adequate resources are available and to help other families understand mental illness. Finally, family members who have suffered the trauma of this illness often need some aspect of renewal either through their own support systems or from the care system.

Families are powerful advocates and can integrate their activities with others so as to play a more effective role. By allying with service user groups, providers and public funders, they can be effective in the political arena. Family members can also be effective in educating the public and with the media in attacking the stigma and lack of knowledge about mental illness.

The community

Changes in the community are more difficult and more long-term in nature. Yet if we wish to ensure that a mental health care system is actually community-based, it is indispensable to work towards community recovery and inclusion.

Community recovery begins when the community and its leaders understand both the effects of mental illness and the societal impact of not delivering effective, efficient services. Recovery begins in earnest when the community and its leaders find ways to harness the potential contribution of service users in every aspect of community life. Stimulating community recovery will involve long-term strategies, the results of which may take decades to realise.

 © THE SAINSBURY CENTRE FOR MENTAL HEALTH, 2002

To secure jobs for service users who have serious mental illnesses and use long-term supports has always been a formidable challenge. Employers and housing owners will be provoked into good practice when they see community leaders such as politicians, educators, clergy, corporate executives and physicians support efforts to help people recover from mental illness and engage in the life of the community.

A vital change that needs to occur within the community is increased services integration. Many people with mental health problems need to access services offered by a variety of public and private providers. For communities to offer the most efficient and effective service, service users must be able to access services rapidly.

Mental health systems must develop strong partnerships with all other social, health and public support systems. A primary responsibility of the mental health provider is to develop long-term plans to work on relationships with other service organisations that will translate into shared care plans and shared resources.

Key points

- 'What providers have traditionally designed are services, rather than a comprehensive community support system that assists service users to achieve the outcomes that they want.' How can you help planners to hold on to the big picture?
- How well does your assessment system meet the four fundamental requirements of (a) focus on individual strength; (b) acknowledgement and encouragement of individual responsibility; (c) self determination and (d) individual need for a life purpose and meaning?
- What is available locally to support families to 'go through their own recovery process'?

 © THE SAINSBURY CENTRE FOR MENTAL HEALTH, 2002

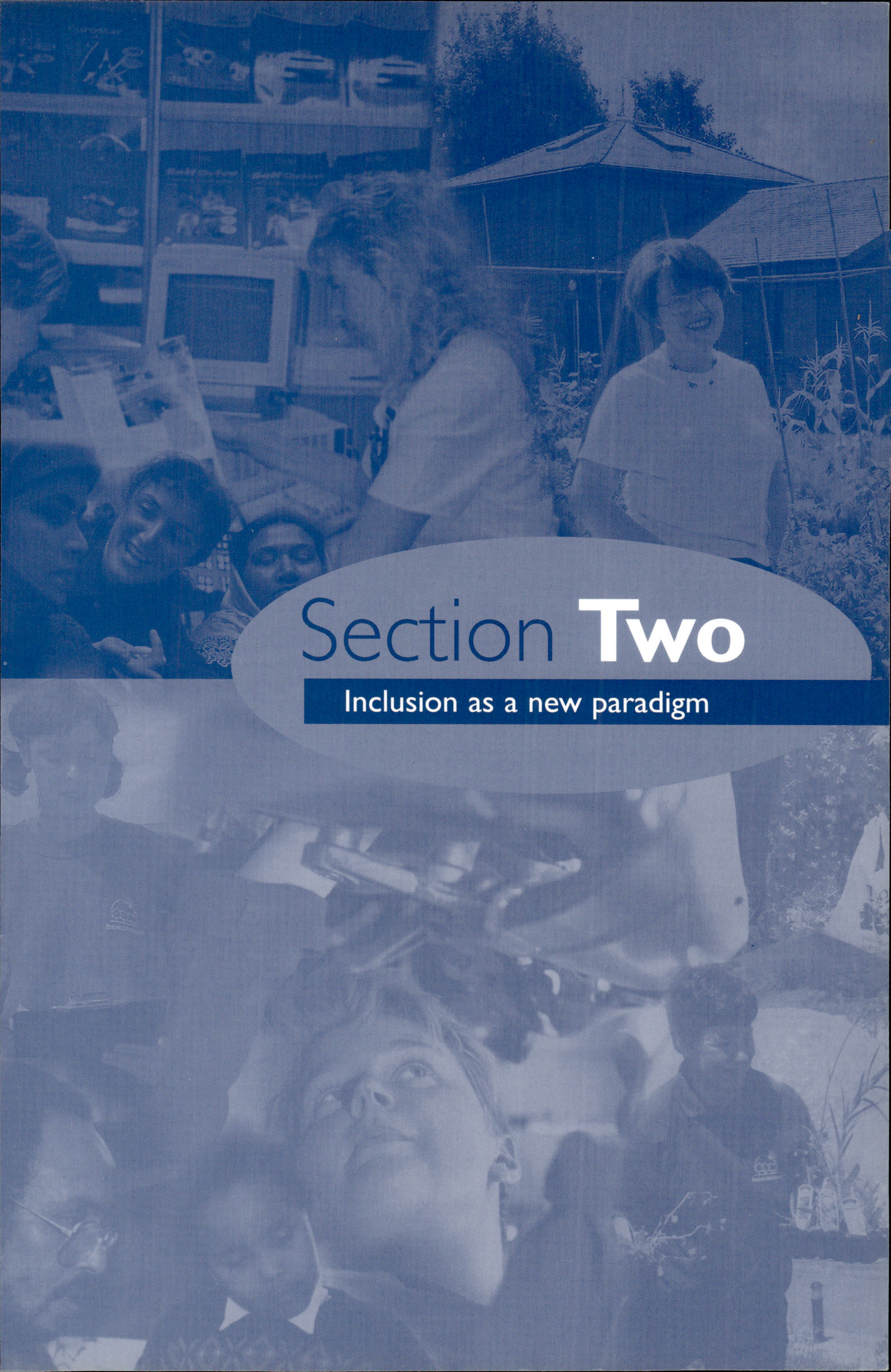

Section Two

Inclusion as a new paradigm

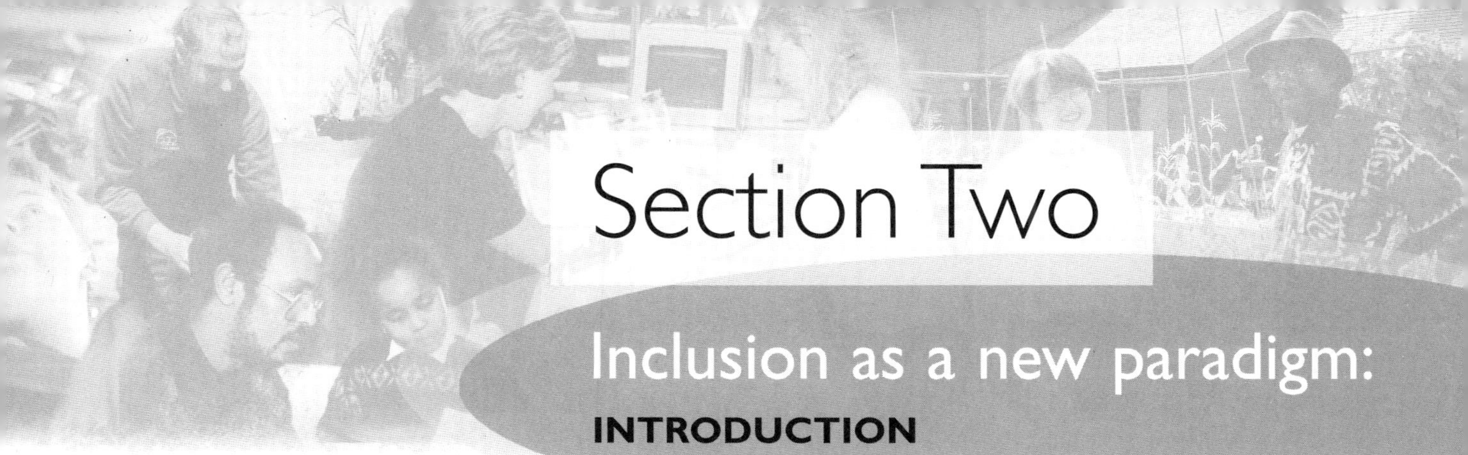

Section Two

Inclusion as a new paradigm: INTRODUCTION

Peter Bates

In the last section we explored some of the things that might be meant by inclusion and community as well as the impact that these ideas might have on mental health services. But why is there currently such a pool of interest in social inclusion and mental health? This section identifies a number of the streams that have fed this pool.

In *Politics and Social Exclusion*, Jon Hyslop and Ann Jackson take us back to the late 1980s and trace the political ideas that have impacted on mental health services in the last decade or so. Consumerism and community care, the underclass and the third way, disability rights and user participation have all shaped our current services. Sometimes these influences have harmonised with each other, while at other times mental health has been an arena of conflict. For example, community care has been perceived as in collision with the public safety agenda.

The next article, *Partnerships for Inclusion* takes us from the national policy agenda to the detail of one locality. The New Labour government's interest in 'joined-up thinking' or improved collaboration between agencies is an important influence on the social inclusion agenda. This article illustrates how a large group of individuals worked together in Bromley to create networks between service users and providers, different mental health services and the wider community.

Fabian Davis reflects on what we can learn from hospital closure in the next article. While most Victorian psychiatric hospitals have now disappeared in England, the transformation has left a lot of unfinished work. People who had lived their whole adult lives in the hospital moved into ordinary houses and their quality of life improved. However, the improvement was often limited as it became clear that their new status of neighbour and fellow shopper did not always generate social networks and meaningful roles.

While friendship does not qualify for a place in this section as a major topic that has influenced policy and practice in the mental health world, it is so pervasive as to justify some attention.

 © THE SAINSBURY CENTRE FOR MENTAL HEALTH, 2002

Friendships occur when there is an exchange of practical help, shared company or intimacy (Richardson and Ritchie, 1989). While occasionally developing when people meet in formal relationships (co-worker, relative, carers, student, neighbour and flatmate), these roles alone are insufficient to ensure that friendship actually occurs.

The building blocks of valued interpersonal relationships include: choosing and having the opportunity to meet, sharing in common experiences and activities, continuity, reciprocity, the skills to build and maintain the contact, and a belief that each has something to offer.

It is perhaps the element of choice that marks friendship out as distinctive from more formal roles, enabling aspects of each other's identity to be revealed. Felce (1988) notes that friendships take many forms, and observers should beware of imposing their own interpretation or denigrating contacts which they perceive as merely superficial. This point is emphasised by O'Brien and O'Brien (Amado, 1993) who note that friendships are sometimes invisible to the outside observer. Individuals, whose sole interactions with others are composed of monosyllables or silent co-existence, could be conducting intimate, emotional relationships in their heads and hearts.

Many people are seeking friendship, and so inclusive mental health services need to understand how the political dimensions of friendship are played out and also what actions can be taken to support the progression from isolation to formal roles, from acquaintance to friend, and from friendship to love.

Some people aim to make friends with other service users, while others wish to make connections with people in the wider community. A brief study by Hughes and Walden (1999) illustrates how difficult this can be – a befriending scheme was introduced but this led to withdrawal by other members of the person's social network – in this case befriending led to 'de-friending'. Additionally, service providers need to remember that relationships and friendships are outside their control – they can create opportunities and provide support, but do no more.

The potential for forming friendships and connections between people with mental health difficulties and the wider community is limited by popular images of mental distress. Lynne Friedli and Elizabeth Gale consider how mental health promotion, a requirement of the *National Service Framework for Mental Health*, can impact on that popular perception. Mental health services, in collaboration with others, must work to increase emotional resilience, strengthen communities and challenge discrimination.

In the final article in this section, Liz Sayce moves beyond education about mental health issues to embrace civil rights for people with mental health problems. She shows how the *Disability Discrimination Act 1995* has begun to achieve a change in culture and a gradual acceptance of the right to equal opportunities by people with physical or sensory impairments. In contrast, people with mental health problems have been left behind, and this makes it vital that alliances are strengthened between disability groups and the mental health lobby.

 © THE SAINSBURY CENTRE FOR MENTAL HEALTH, 2002

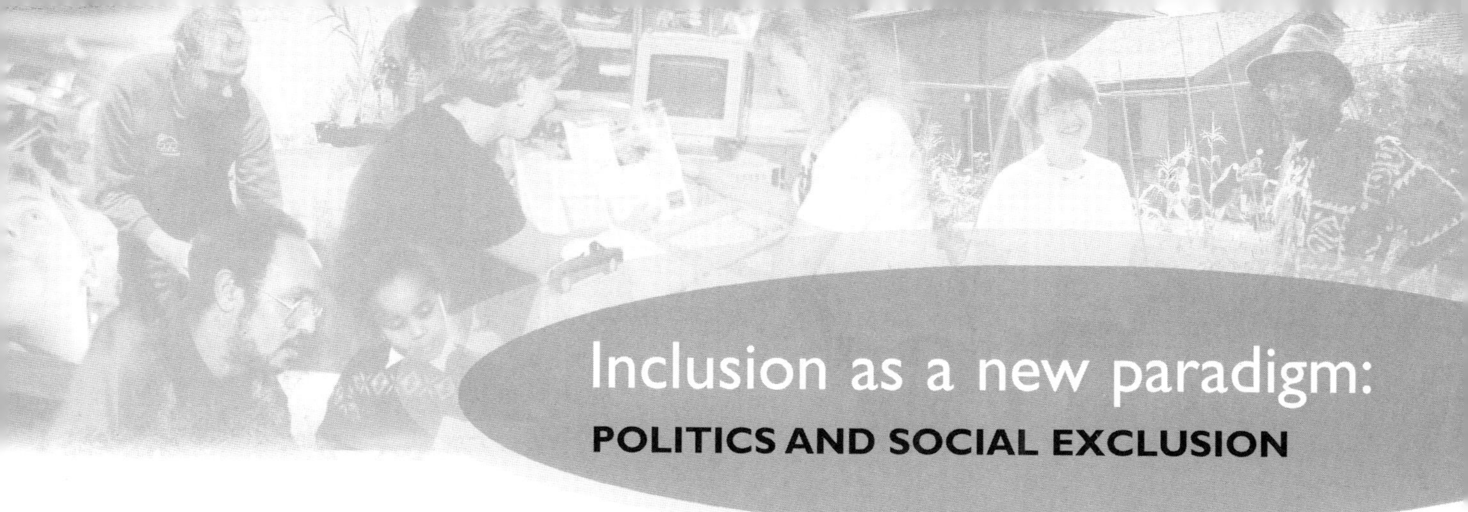

Inclusion as a new paradigm:
POLITICS AND SOCIAL EXCLUSION

LIBRARY
CHARLES FRE CAMPUS
DE MONTFORT UNIVERSITY

Jon Hyslop and Ann Jackson

At a first glance, it can appear that the policies of successive governments on mental health issues have borne no particular relationship to the main political agendas of the Conservative and Labour Parties. However, a closer examination will reveal that mental health policy is as much driven by ideology as the wider fields of health, education and employment. Over the last decade (and particularly since the election of New Labour in 1997), the social exclusion/social inclusion debate has made a particularly significant impact. This chapter attempts to set the social policy context for some of the issues and practices examined in greater detail later on.

The Conservative Party agenda for mental health: 1987–1997

Community care as consumerism

From within the mental health field, it is possible to trace a history of community care that completely ignores party politics. At first glance, this history can seem like an inevitable progression from the discovery of and widespread use of anti-psychotic drugs during the 1950s through the anti-psychiatry movement in the 1960s, to the hospital scandals of the 1970s and the Griffiths Report of the late 80s (Griffiths, 1988).

The White Paper preceding the *NHS and Community Care Act 1990*, (Department of Health, 1988) explicitly locates the emerging policy within this history. However, there is another history, less frequently discussed by those within the mental health field. Very unusually, the Community Care Act was preceded by two White Papers: the second – *Working for Patients* (Department of Health, 1989) is explicit in its consumerist ideology.

At the 1987 Conservative Party Conference, health secretary John Moore had proposed to reduce taxation for people with private health insurance – effectively allowing better off people to opt out of the NHS. The public backlash was immediate, and it was rumoured that even Prime Minister Margaret Thatcher thought he had gone too far: she replaced Moore with Kenneth Clarke, and commissioned a review of the NHS.

 © THE SAINSBURY CENTRE FOR MENTAL HEALTH, 2002

The *Prime Minister's Review* recommended setting up an 'internal market' by splitting the service into purchasers, such as health authorities, and providers (new independently managed hospital trusts) which would compete with one another for business. This would allow new private hospitals to compete with the NHS for public money, effectively beginning the privatisation from the supply end. It was Clarke's stroke of brilliance to combine this internal market policy with community care, with the latter agenda helping to ensure the co-operation of health and social care professions (Paton, 1990).

Community care: more choice for mental health service users?

While it had always been true that the vast majority of people with diagnosed mental health problems lived outside a hospital setting most of the time, the focus had always been on what happened in hospital (for example, the *Mental Health Act 1983* virtually ignored treatment outside hospital). The new community care policy promised a much-improved range of non-hospital services.

Perhaps the most ambitious of these new processes was care management. Instead of being tied to a fixed pattern of local provision, each local social services department employed care managers who had access to a flexible budget, which could be used to support a 'client' (not patient) in whatever way seemed most appropriate. This offered a much wider potential for people labelled as mentally ill to be supported in engaging with their communities than had previously existed.

A similar development from within the hospital system was the care programme approach (CPA), (DoH, 1990), in which clients and keyworkers collaborated to produce an agreed plan of care to be carried out by a multi-disciplinary team. This 'enforced discharge planning' (Leff, 1997) was largely a response to a series of high profile media stories of 'failed' care in the community (Muijen, 1997).

However well intended, these two processes were complicated (and arguably compromised) by the fact that care management was operated within social services and CPA within health authorities, with separate professional, managerial and budgetary responsibility. In many areas, the inability of health and social services managers to negotiate joint working arrangements delayed the implementation of both initiatives, and compromised their effectiveness.

Budgets both for care managers and the services they offered were tightly squeezed throughout the early 1990s, meaning that staff had few choices to offer besides those they could supply themselves, or that had been paid for in advance by local health and social services. Similarly, care management was available to progressively fewer people, as service criteria were limited to those perceived as having 'severe and enduring' mental health problems, again limiting the choice supposedly improved through consumerism.

 © THE SAINSBURY CENTRE FOR MENTAL HEALTH, 2002

Whilst people generally felt they had more choice outside hospital than in (Carpenter and Sbaraini, 1997), there were definite limits to the perceived extent of integration with the community. According to one survey (Rose, 1996) feeling lonely was the second largest 'daily hassle' faced by service users in the community.

> "*Wanting more contacts in a community which doesn't want contact with you is, not surprisingly, associated with discontent.*" (Rose, 1996)

Despite their relocation from hospital, mental health services remained largely treatment-focused, and failed to grapple effectively with the less straightforward issue of participation.

Consumer choice: how far did it really go?

There were other limitations: for one thing, the budgets were devolved to professionals, not service users. To some extent, this was remedied by direct payments. The *Community Care (Direct Payments) Act 1996* gives local authorities the power to make cash payments for community care direct to individuals who need services. This was the last major piece of disability legislation introduced by the last Conservative government which suffered a landslide defeat in a general election shortly after the Act came into effect in the spring of 1997. However, the law continues to be firmly supported by the new administration despite (or perhaps because of) its free market credentials.

The origins of social exclusion: Charles Murray and the underclass

In the late 1980s and early 1990s, the concept of an 'underclass' came into the mainstream UK politics. Imported from America by Charles Murray (Murray, 1990), the underclass was represented as a section of the population bound into a trans-generational cycle of poverty and dependence on the state largely through its own fecklessness and inability to accept responsibility.

The central difference between the underclass and older concepts of poverty was the location of the responsibility within the individual, through a series of linked self-perpetuating behaviours (unemployment, drug use, crime and family breakdown) (Anderson, 2000). For the Conservative Party, the single mother was adopted as a symbol of the relationship between immorality and social breakdown. Although the 'mentally ill' weren't explicitly located within the underclass, many of the related policies (such as tightening entitlement to benefits and other withdrawals of resources) had a direct impact.

 © THE SAINSBURY CENTRE FOR MENTAL HEALTH, 2002

New Labour: 1997–2001

The underclass and the third way

The traditional Labour perspective on the responsibility for poverty, of course, was very different to that of the Conservatives. It was seen as the responsibility of a socialist government to assist the victims of capitalism by transferring resources from business and the well-off. However, after four successive general election defeats, the Labour Party desperately needed a more voter-friendly approach.

The huge benefits bill and the taxation needed to pay it had been a critical factor in Margaret Thatcher's election in 1979, and the perception of Labour as a 'tax and spend' party was seen as an electoral liability (Ellison and Pearson, 1998). The concept of an underclass and the related process of social exclusion consequently had some appeal.

Whilst New Labour did not accept the blaming of the underclass for its own circumstances, it did substantially accept the behavioural mechanisms by which the underclass was supposed to sustain itself. It then became the responsibility of individuals to help themselves out of poverty and the responsibility of government to provide the opportunities for them to do so, rather than to accept responsibility and compensate them. This 'third way' can be seen in the following quote from then shadow-Chancellor Gordon Brown:

> *"I am proud that we have an agenda for political reform which means that we can extend opportunities to participate to people who have never had them or to whom they are not available at the moment ... What we should do is maximise opportunities that are available for education, employment, culture and politics."*
> (Gordon Brown profiled in *Community Care*, 17–23 October 1996)

Labour, social exclusion and Europe

Whereas the outgoing Thatcherites had looked to America for their inspiration, New Labour looked to Europe. In 1992 and 1993, European Commission policy documents began to refer increasingly to the concept of social exclusion, and what could be done to minimise it (Stevens, Bur and Young, 2000).

The lack of clarity around the meaning of the term, which remains a feature of the inclusion/exclusion debate today, can be seen simultaneously as a strength and weakness. On the plus side, it has been applied to a much wider range of circumstances than words like 'poverty' and 'the poor' describe, and can therefore be seen as 'holistic'. On the minus side, it can be interpreted in such a wide variety of different manners that it risks losing meaning.

 © THE SAINSBURY CENTRE FOR MENTAL HEALTH, 2002

The New Deal: a holistic approach?

Despite these broader concepts of exclusion, the main area outside mental health services in which the government seems keen to encourage participation of people labelled as mentally ill is the labour market.

Soon after the new government began its tenure "it identified disability benefits as the target of reforming cost cuts" (Barkham, 2000) focusing on the Disability Living Allowance and Invalid Care Allowance. Both of these benefits were framed initially in terms of physical disability, making it hard for people with mental health needs to claim, and making them especially vulnerable to the 'proposed new assessment' process.

At the same time the government began its New Deal. While the scheme provides a number of welcome initiatives for people willing and able to work, it did little to counter the well-known structural barriers to employment (potential loss of benefits, inflexible working hours etc), (Roulstone, 2000).

The New Deal locates the problem of unemployment within the 'mentally ill' person; risking increasing stigma and lowering self-esteem for those who 'fail' to help themselves.

When it is considered that a mere 13% of people with a severe mental health problem are in employment (Sayce, 1998) the scale of this risk becomes apparent. If work is the only available and socially valid source of income, the resultant economic powerlessness of people with mental health problems is likely to remain a major factor in social exclusion. Unemployment then is:

> *"To lose one's credibility as a human agent and citizen. Being poor then adds insult to this injury."* (Pilgrim & Waldron, 1998).

Disability rights in Britain and Europe

The creation of a Disability Rights Commission in April 2000 has been a response to some of these criticisms. The Commission's stated objective is to promote equality of opportunity and eliminate discrimination, utilising both *The Disability Discrimination Act 1995* and the European rights incorporated into UK law by *The Human Rights Act 1998*. These European rights have themselves been strengthened by the *1999 Amsterdam Treaty*, which explicitly empowers EU member states to take action to combat discrimination based on disability (see ***Section Five***).

 © THE SAINSBURY CENTRE FOR MENTAL HEALTH, 2002

Participation and citizenship

Social exclusion is supposed to be a process as well as an outcome (Anderson, 2000). Policies and schemes to increase participation and reduce exclusion often operate at both levels (i.e. they aim to promote participation of excluded groups in the process of change, as well as promoting greater participation in society as a final outcome).

Recent government health (and mental health) policy has stressed the desirability of including service users in the process of developing and running services. The *National Service Framework for Mental Health* and its precursor, *Modernising Mental Health Services: Safe Sound and Supportive* both repeatedly mention 'user involvement' and 'user participation' as desirable and even necessary (Department of Health, 1998b; Department of Health, 1999b).

However, at the same time as advancing participation, the state also appears to want to increase the degree of compulsion and control available to professionals. The White Paper *Reforming The Mental Health Act* proposes new powers for compulsory treatment outside hospitals, and the indefinite detention of people on the basis of perceived dangerousness (Department of Health & Home Office, 2000).

Peck (2000) describes the apparent contradictions in terms of tensions between the 'head' and 'heart' of government. On the one hand the modernisation agenda claims to promote participation in policy-making (pluralist heart) and on the other imposes (centralist head) policy, prior to the completion of a full consultation process.

This type of conflict has also been observed in the wider European context. Participation at a policy level is organised from the top down, usually as a specific means to an end. It is policy-makers who dictate the terms of such participation. In the terms of the 'active citizenship' model with which participation is often identified, the power-holders are prepared to devolve the responsibilities without devolving the rights. If participation is to be anything other than tokenism and manipulation, then it must allow for outcomes other than those dictated by policy makers (Stevens, Bur and Young, 2000).

There is some evidence that European policies are taking this point on board. For example, the new 'equal' initiative stresses the importance of citizen participation in the design and evaluation of community-based initiatives, as well as in their delivery. It is this European money that is making possible some of the more imaginative approaches to community involvement.

© THE SAINSBURY CENTRE FOR MENTAL HEALTH, 2002

Summary

Throughout the late 1980s and early 1990s, the focus of mental health services switched from hospital to community, from patients to consumers. While these changes resulted in a greater degree of freedom and control over treatment, they substantially failed to facilitate greater community integration. Resources remained in the hands of professionals, and mental ill-health was associated with dangerousness in the public imagination, resulting in greater stigma and isolation for people labelled as mentally ill.

Pilgrim and Waldron (1998) have suggested that the move from the old institution to the community has been incomplete, and has resulted in a continuing emphasis on buildings and professional practices, that they call 're-institutionalisation'. They argue that this policy trend has not resulted in 'citizenship of service users in genuine community settings'.

Since New Labour came to power, there has also been a shift in the conceptualisation of participation, mirroring a pan-European debate on the role of the citizen in the state. However, participation has been narrowly defined, typically in terms of participation in the labour market, or participation in the planning and delivery of mental health services. Simultaneously, the government has sought to allay public fears relating to 'dangerous' people with mental health problems by proposing greater powers of compulsion and control, and emphasising the primacy of public safety over other issues (e.g. *Safety First*, Department of Health, 2001a).

More positively, both British and European policy has recently made significant progress towards ensuring the rights of disabled people are enforceable, particularly within the employment field. European and UK funding initiatives are more focused on involving citizens than ever before.

The UK government with the creation of the influential Social Exclusion Unit has signalled a commitment to 'joined up thinking'. Both funding and policy-making now favours initiatives that involve service users and cross service boundaries. Arguably, the ground has been well prepared for a fundamental re-think in the way in which people labelled as 'mentally ill' are included in society.

 © THE SAINSBURY CENTRE FOR MENTAL HEALTH, 2002

Key points

In your locality...

- Do mental health services reach the right people?
- Is care provided in creative and individualised ways? Are direct payments easily available?
- How are mental health services working with others to combat 'poor skills, low incomes, poor housing, bad health and family breakdown'?
- Are service users involved in (a) the design and delivery of mental health services, and (b) decision making in the local community?

 © THE SAINSBURY CENTRE FOR MENTAL HEALTH, 2002

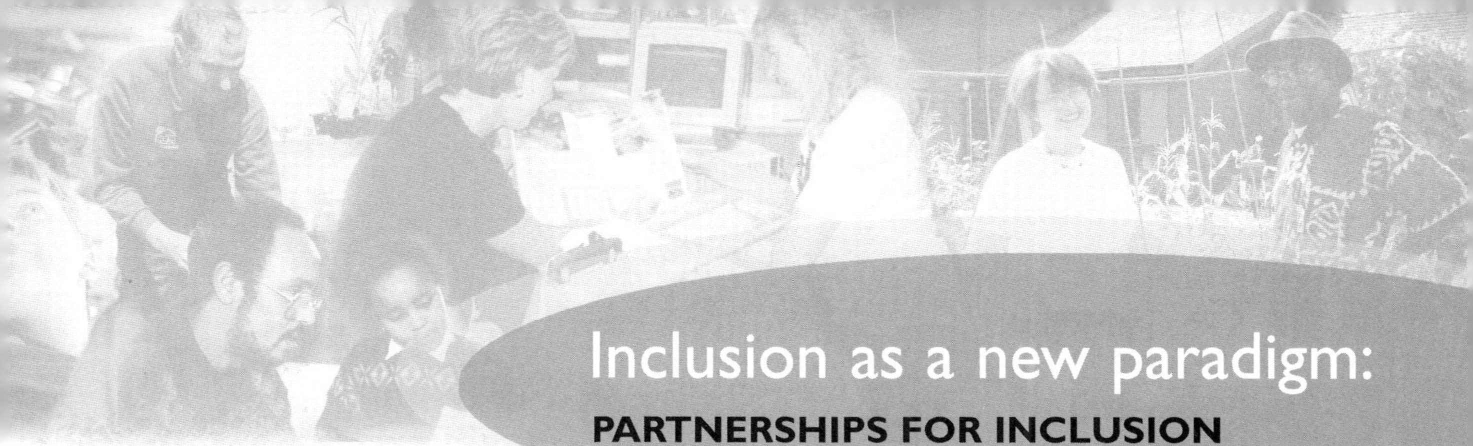

Inclusion as a new paradigm:

PARTNERSHIPS FOR INCLUSION

Roy Batten, Pam Buttrey, Jon Cribbens, Fabian A. Davis, Michael Fletcher, Louise Holden, Phil Jones, Iain Kitchener, Helen Macklin, Kim Minter, Kevin Pace, Karen Pavey, Nikki Slater and Richard K. Sutton.

Partnerships between service users and providers

The District Rehabilitation Service in Bromley, South East London, began to focus on user involvement in the early 1990s. Service user organisations were involved in staff recruitment, a user consultant was appointed on an honorary contract and users had a substantial input to evaluation of services.

One key output was the development of a user satisfaction survey that enables the service to gather evidence on its own practice. The assessment criteria illustrated emerged from the content analysis of forty interviews (see user satisfaction questionnaire) with service users who explained what they found valuable about a good quality rehabilitation service (Bond and Davis, 1997). Maintaining this level of accountability to the people who use the service is vital in the development of a partnership relationship. An informal user group was established from this to guide staff in their future work.

 © THE SAINSBURY CENTRE FOR MENTAL HEALTH, 2002

User satisfaction questionnaire

Please tick which of the following best describes the service you receive from the community rehabilitation service:

	Strongly agree	*Agree*	*Disagree*	*Strongly disagree*
Easy to make contact with	☐	☐	☐	☐
Good relationship with keyworker	☐	☐	☐	☐
Enough time with staff	☐	☐	☐	☐
Available on a regular and continuous basis	☐	☐	☐	☐
Have trust and confidentiality	☐	☐	☐	☐
Good at listening/giving advice	☐	☐	☐	☐
Help with emotional concerns	☐	☐	☐	☐
Help with practical matters	☐	☐	☐	☐
They respect your opinions	☐	☐	☐	☐

© THE SAINSBURY CENTRE FOR MENTAL HEALTH, 2002

Partnership with the whole mental health community

In 1997 three local, long-term intervention teams took over from the district rehabilitation service, working with everyone with a long-term mental health problem, not just people moving out of hospital and those in supported accommodation.

This enlarged the service by over three-fold and made local community partnerships a more realistic possibility than operating at a district wide level for a small percentage of the people in need. It seemed like the right time to introduce a local values framework to support the wider development of socially inclusive practice in partnership with local community organisations.

We wanted to capture some of the principles embedded in the local experience gained over the last ten years and to codify the evidence base derived from the literature. It was also important as the service became more competent at supporting social inclusion that it have a position on and a strategy to deal with the forces of social devaluation and exclusion.

To do this it seemed that a clarification of the local values base was a pre-requisite to the development of any service philosophy, so a values framework (Turner-Crowson, 1997) was developed as follows:

We wanted to

- combat stigma;
- agree a statement of mission and values;
- stimulate service improvements linked by these common values to a shared purpose.

How we did it

- We began with a group made up of equal numbers of service users, providers, purchasers and carers.
- We linked up with the local joint strategic planning group.
- It took over a year and culminated in a large consensus conference where over 100 people representing 20 organisations agreed the mission and values statement.

 ©THE SAINSBURY CENTRE FOR MENTAL HEALTH, 2002

What does the mission and values statement say?

- The mission is: 'To promote recovery and a valued lifestyle in the community'.
- The values for purchasers cover access, equity, comprehensiveness and consultation.
- The values for practitioners include respectful relationships, choice, community partnership, collaborative approaches and positive imagery.

Have new services developed?

- Service users are involved in the local NHS trust as consultant advisors in one of the new long-term intervention teams.
- Service users are represented at the NHS trust head office.
- The clubhouse has influenced the recruitment and retention policies of a large national employer.
- A local long-term intervention team, all the residential care services and the outreach service, serving 250 people, have adopted person-centred planning (see ***Section Six***).
- Some service users, their friends and allies have joined together in a 'circle of friends' – a structured way of working together to help someone to achieve their ambitions (Bates, 2000).

Partnerships with the wider community

When the long-term intervention teams were set up locally it quickly became apparent there was indeed a considerable amount of unmet need in the user population.

We elaborated the service philosophy into a set of detailed goals, and then into an assessment tool (see ***Section Five***) and the questionnaire was used to make a detailed study of the support needs of the users in one of the teams. The results revealed the expected pattern of relatively good physical integration with social integration lagging far behind.

In other words, service users were using general community buildings, but most of their relationships were still with other service users. As a result of this survey, conducted in 1999, the Developing Valued Lifestyles Project (DeVeLoP) was established to support further work on social inclusion in one of the long-term intervention teams.

DeVeLoP is a collaboration between the long-term intervention team, a clubhouse, a group of service user consultants, the local user group, the local advocacy service, Mind and a community housing association providing residential care and an outreach service.

 © THE SAINSBURY CENTRE FOR MENTAL HEALTH, 2002

The DeVeLoP steering group supports and guides the long-term intervention team and has three tasks. Firstly, the group stops mental health services 'doing social inclusion to people' by virtue of its mixed membership but shared principles. Secondly, it is a resource to care co-ordinators and service users in accessing local resources or dealing with discrimination and stigma. Thirdly, the group keeps local people abreast of the issues faced by those with mental health problems in recovering and leading valued lives in the community by holding a monthly education and networking forum in ordinary community venues.

The focus of the project is to promote and support person-centred planning. This will develop and maximise service users' access to:

- mainstream community facilities;
- impartial information on which to base decisions;
- ordinary and valued relationships and respect;
- social inclusion and involvement in community life;
- financial, physical and mental health support.

There are direct links from this membership to local networks such as LETS (Local Exchange Trading Schemes), the local business community, chamber of commerce and several religious communities.

Formal links to mainstream education and leisure resources are currently under discussion. Many informal links already exist through the project membership and through the community outreach activities of team members. Service users and care co-ordinators are actively developing plans for increasing opportunities for social inclusion.

Conclusion

All three kinds of partnership are needed if people with mental health problems are to be fully empowered and included in their communities. Each mental health service must involve its users, build relationships with other mental health service providers and link strongly with non-mental health networks in the community. Building all these connections around a strong focus on person-centred planning ensures that time and effort is devoted to the right things and also safeguards the process from 'doing inclusion to people'.

 © THE SAINSBURY CENTRE FOR MENTAL HEALTH, 2002

Key points

In Bromley...

- Users defined the criteria against which service quality was monitored.
- A wide range of mental health agencies developed a shared vision for supporting people to have a meaningful life in the community.
- A group has taken on the specific task of challenging discrimination and educating local people about mental health services.

© THE SAINSBURY CENTRE FOR MENTAL HEALTH, 2002

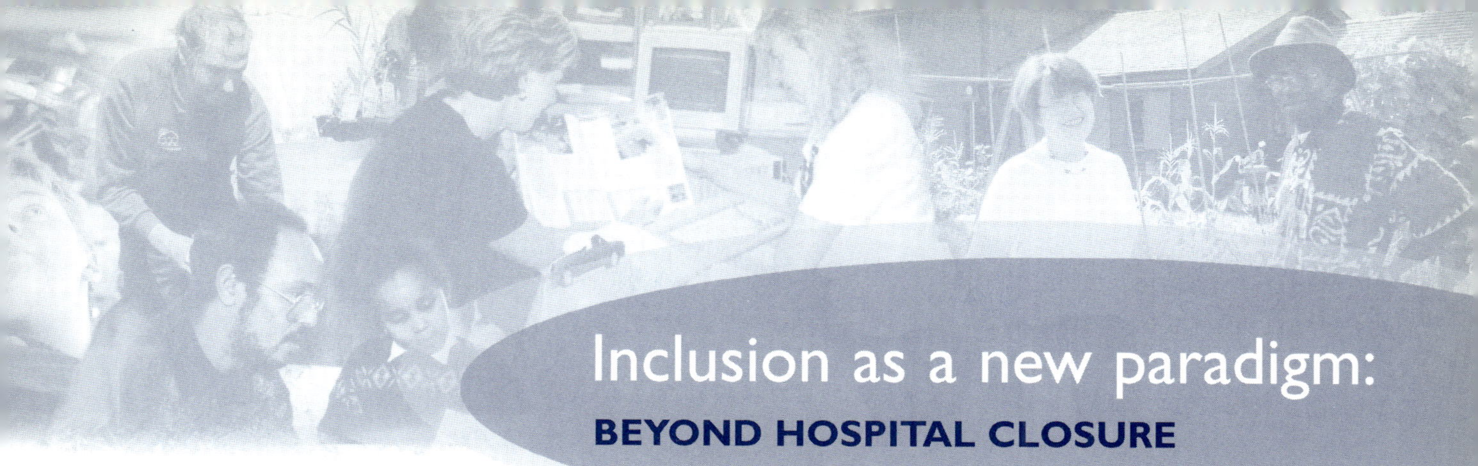

Inclusion as a new paradigm:
BEYOND HOSPITAL CLOSURE

Fabian A. Davis

The Positive Futures Programme

In early 1988 a small multi-disciplinary resettlement team was brought together by a south east London mental health service to help those people in a large and distant Victorian asylum move back home. A new team of staff was recruited to work with the hospital nursing team.

This brought a new perspective to the resettlement process – one of community integration rather than re-provision. This was based on the new staff's previous experience of hospital closure and of supporting people in their own homes, combined with the social model of disability and information gleaned from learning disability services. The team also noticed that the notion of community integration had been marginalised in the past and set out to include senior management, service users and carers in all their work right from the start.

The Positive Futures Programme, as it was named by Bromley User Group, became a £35m project for Bromley Health Authority. The programme ran over four years and involved several other district services which spent similar sums. Positive Futures planned and implemented new services previously provided at Cane Hill and Oakwood Hospitals in Surrey and Kent respectively.

From 1988–1992 the resettlement team led clinical practice at the hospital and the development of new services in the community, in partnership with hospital management and a project development team. By taking on a positive role in caretaking the old service and developing the architecture of the new they formed a bridge between the hospital and the community both for staff and residents.

The team involved staff from grass roots to director level in the planning of new services through a wide-ranging system of inter-linked functional working groups. Allied to this was its commitment to user and carer participation in the development process. To this end it brought together residents' families on a regular basis in conference format (with cream teas) to look at the process of community return and the kinds of service models being proposed. The families felt genuinely involved and supported by the openness and clarity of purpose with which these tasks were conducted.

To foster user involvement the focus was on choice, decision making, and understanding who residents had been and were now, in relation to their lives in the community. This meant working resolutely to create circumstances within the hospital that mirrored the new arrangements and taking enough time to allow people to make informed choices about where and with whom they were going to live.

As the programme progressed the team increased the level of user participation to the extent that potential residents were able to be involved in advising on difficult purchasing preferences. At a more personal level residents were enabled to buy belongings and furnishings for their new homes within predefined budgetary limits.

Person-centred planning, based on O'Brien's 'five accomplishments' (O'Brien, 1987), became the approach used to help people develop their lives once the physical moves were achieved (see ***Section Six***). Person-centred planning in mental health was first publicised in the UK as *Getting to Know You* (Thomas and Rose, 1986; Thomas *et al.*, 1990). Clinical budgets and trust funds were brought together to allow financial flexibility (resulting in something akin to direct payments) that supported personal choices.

The success of the programme can be evidenced by the change in plans that resulted from the above processes. In 1987 the plans were for all residents to go to 12-bedded hostels or to alternative hospital facilities. By 1990 these plans came to fruition in a much modified form. The programme included the purchase of nine five-bedroom and two five-bedroom (plus two-bed flat) houses. There were also two ten-bedroom nursing homes, one for frail older people and one for people with challenging behaviour, a clubhouse, two mental health centres, an extension to a third centre, the provision of two day centres and two ten-bed hospital units. Since 1990, this network of provision has been further modified to individualise provision still further.

All these new facilities used existing buildings which were refurbished to a high standard in keeping with the nature of their tasks, either ordinary domestic or work oriented (Braisby *et al.*, 1988). They were all in safe and attractive neighbourhoods close to centres of population well served with community facilities. Houses were in residential areas and the clubhouse and day centres were close to industrial or retail areas.

What about the evidence base?

The team began with a limited knowledge of published research that supported their approach and at the time much of the available material was from America. It was only during and after the Positive Futures Programme that a more concerted effort was made to scour the literature. The search is summarised here and, on the whole, it supports the Positive Futures approach.

 © THE SAINSBURY CENTRE FOR MENTAL HEALTH, 2002

The evidence for better living in the community: housing issues

Socially inclusive mental health practices like those described above seek to promote physical and social integration by enabling people to live in culturally valued accommodation and so gain a culturally valued lifestyle.

Physical integration occurs when people with mental health problems live amongst other citizens, rather than in separate specialised places, while social integration occurs when a person with mental health difficulties counts valued citizens as the majority of people in their circle of acquaintances, friends and loved ones. Positive outcomes are related to doing the ordinary things in life in ways that most people prefer.

In supported housing, the number of people in the home (Hull and Thomson, 1981), and their proximity and access to ordinary community facilities (Canadian Council on Social Development, 1986), are paramount. More 'independent' small homes in high quality houses in middle income communities with more accessible social activities are most effective at supporting social inclusion (Cournos, 1987).

But to make this work staff must respect people by supporting their dignity, self-esteem and reputation whilst avoiding over-protection and restriction. They must pay active attention to enabling people to engage in valued life activities and pursuits. Such environmental factors contribute more to the success or failure of socially inclusive outcomes than an individual resident's personal characteristics or mental state (Hull and Thomson, 1981).

People leaving hospital like ordinary housing (Knapp *et al.*, 1992), feel less controlled, and develop complex social networks (Anderson *et al.*, 1993). They also find education and religion, then living circumstances, health, social relations, and work, leisure and family relations more satisfying (Dansereau *et al.*, 1990). People get anxious on moving from institutions but this feeling subsides. People's community skills improve and there are transient increases in domestic skills (Leff, 1995) on moving to supported homes in the community. In short, positive symptoms remain stable and negative symptoms improve.

It takes time for ordinary social networks to develop. Sokolovsky *et al.* (1978) concluded that people with schizophrenia with extensive and complex social networks were at lower risk of relapse. Having a confidant is well documented as protective against depression (Brown & Harris, 1978). Anderson *et al.*, (1993) found more friends in the social networks of psychiatric hospital leavers in supported housing than matched 'stayers'. One year gains were sustained with more confidants emerging in years one to five (Leff, 1995).

Living in ordinary housing increases satisfaction with services (Knapp *et al.*, 1992; Anderson *et al.*, 1993). Service users prefer living in existing housing, as long as it is in good condition, to specialised accommodation. Self-contained independent living with support brought in is

 © THE SAINSBURY CENTRE FOR MENTAL HEALTH, 2002

generally preferred to residential care with live in staff (Tanzman, 1993). On the other hand individualisation at the expense of sharing with friends or loved ones is not valued.

As might be expected physical integration is usually more advanced than social integration (Dansereau *et al.*, 1990). Dependence on staff increases with house size and staff of smaller houses make more effort at establishing resident independence (Knapp *et al.*, 1992). Despite this even some physically better integrated houses remain socially distant because of task centred, hierarchical atmospheres with staff fostering dependence rather than a social, emotional and democratic partnership resulting in adult interdependence and reciprocity (Golden, 1982).

Having the same variety and choices in life as valued citizens counts for much in terms of the identity of people who rely on mental health services. It is important however to recognise that while trying to develop a level playing field for people at risk of social exclusion it is also important to try and expand the range of what count as culturally valued roles and activities. Freeing people from a reliance on internalised social norms and ideals based on service preconceptions of normality goes a long way to enabling people who have had mental health problems to feel less guilty about how they live and what they do (Davis, 2001).

Work issues

The presence or absence of work has serious implications for all. People without employment are much more likely to be clinically depressed and use mental health services. Work has a powerful impact on self-image, social identity, status, role and life meaning (Smith, 1985). Without work all this suffers. For people with severe mental health problems, the value of supported open employment in culturally valued settings has been demonstrated (Bond *et al.*, 1997). 'Place and train' work schemes are superior to more traditional sheltered 'train and place' schemes (Crowther *et al.*, 2000). For a fuller description of work issues see ***Section Three***.

Conclusion

In many parts of the United Kingdom, the Victorian psychiatric hospital has been closed for a decade. People now want individualised living arrangements, participation in the community on their own terms and meaningful daytime occupation. These factors all affect mental health outcomes. These studies also challenge contemporary commissioners to found services upon a sound evidence base. The old hospitals may have closed but transformation is not complete.

 © THE SAINSBURY CENTRE FOR MENTAL HEALTH, 2002

Key points

- Is service design based on a thorough knowledge of the available research?
- Do people live in safe and attractive neighbourhoods well served with community facilities?
- What is being done to support service users in developing social networks with citizens outside the mental health community?
- Are your residential units too big?
- How are residential care staff trained to promote independence and community participation?
- What efforts have been made to encourage specific community audiences to be welcoming of difference?

 © THE SAINSBURY CENTRE FOR MENTAL HEALTH, 2002

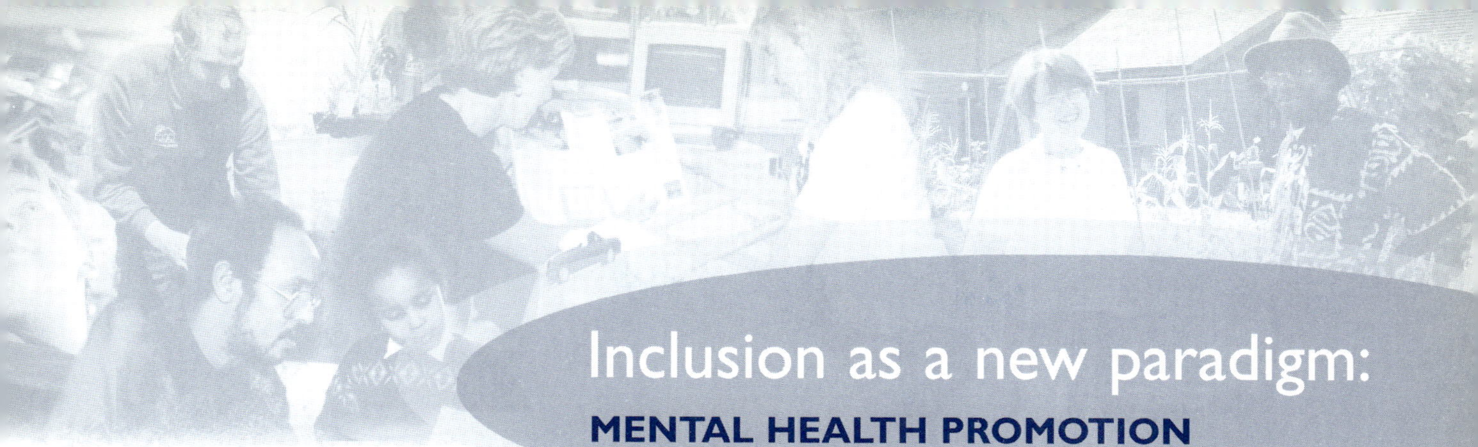

Inclusion as a new paradigm: MENTAL HEALTH PROMOTION

Lynne Friedli and Elizabeth Gale

> *"Of course, social inclusion is very New Labour, very National Service Framework in fact. The problem is, what are the values underpinning this interest in tackling social exclusion and who is going to have to change? Will it be the people who manage the excluding (exclusion is never accidental – on the contrary, it is painstakingly planned, managed, implemented and protected), or will it be the excluded doing a bit of transformation?*
>
> *"It's an uncomfortable fact that throughout history, people have been 'left out' for a very good reason – that to allow them in – women, gays, black people, the mad – is seriously disruptive to 'the way we do things round here'."* (Notes from our own correspondent: the tea trolley, *Breakthrough*, May/June 2000).

The current commitment to social inclusion provides a significant opportunity for fundamental changes in what it means to experience mental health problems. It offers potential for a new vision of what is meant by mental health services, how and where they are delivered and the relationship between services and service users. At the same time, the eager adoption of concepts of inclusion by the mainstream has led to concerns about whose interests are driving the agenda.

This chapter looks at what mental health promotion can contribute to debates about citizenship and social inclusion and the opportunities presented by Standard One of the *National Service Framework for Mental Health* (mentality/SCMH 2001). It also considers some of the lessons that can be learned from user/survivor perspectives and the importance of addressing the values that underpin strategies to reduce social exclusion.

In some cases, the language of social inclusion can be a way of avoiding more challenging debates about justice, equity and civil liberties. It is in danger of meaning: 'It's our game and we define the rules; we'd like you to join in, but it's still our game'. Social inclusion may be less about re-thinking what it means to be a citizen, and more about offering a reward for conformity.

For users, the social inclusion agenda cannot be separated from the history of mental health service provision and people's individual and collective experiences of coercion and disempowerment. More broadly, we need to tackle the exclusion of users and survivors in the context of other excluded, vilified or marginalised groups: refugees and asylum seekers, young offenders, black men, single mothers.

 © THE SAINSBURY CENTRE FOR MENTAL HEALTH, 2002

Social exclusion and health

It is now widely recognised that social exclusion damages mental and physical health and contributes significantly to health inequalities (Kawachi *et al.*, 1997; Friedli 2000). Research in the field of 'stress biology' demonstrates how experiences associated with exclusion – the chronic stress of racism, injustice, fear of crime, lack of control and perceived powerlessness – impact on the immune system and the cardiovascular system, affecting blood pressure, cholesterol levels, susceptibility to infection and growth in childhood.

How people feel is written on the body and expressed in a wide range of physical health problems (Marmot and Wilkinson, 1999). Of course, on almost any indicator, people with mental health problems are among the most excluded groups and are also at increased risk of physical illness, much of which remains undetected.

Social exclusion is therefore a major public health issue both for excluded populations in general and for those who are excluded as a consequence of their mental illness diagnosis. It is increasingly clear that the erosion of mental, emotional and spiritual well-being is one of the key pathways through which social exclusion damages health.

Mental health impact

Until recently, mental health promotion has been little recognised in debates about mental health. Within the NHS, local priorities have been driven by the need to improve mental health services, with a focus on ensuring that those who are thought to need medical treatment receive it.

While local authorities have taken the lead in many areas that have a strong influence on mental health, notably neighbourhood renewal, an explicit framework for addressing public mental health has been missing. This means that at a strategic level, mental health impact (see **box 1**) is not routinely included as part of the decision making process, with significant consequences for the mental well-being of communities and the quality of life for people with mental health problems.

 © THE SAINSBURY CENTRE FOR MENTAL HEALTH, 2002

BOX 1 Mental health impact assessment

Mental health impact assessment is a way of including mental health in the decision making process. It means that committees, task forces, advisory groups and other forums where decisions are made need to ask 'what impact will this action have on people's mental health?'

Finding answers to this question will mean drawing on many different sources of expertise, including service users, the mental health voluntary sector and public health specialists with an understanding of risk and protective factors for mental health. It will also mean recognising that how people feel is not an abstract and elusive concept, but a significant measure of health and well-being.

National Service Framework: Standard One

Standard One of the *National Service Framework for Mental Health (NSF)* (DoH, 1999b) places mental health promotion firmly on the policy agenda (Department of Health, 2001b). It requires health and social services to promote the mental health of local communities **and** to take action to tackle the discrimination and exclusion experienced by people with mental health problems. This provides a unique opportunity to acknowledge that we all have mental health needs, whether or not we have a diagnosis (see **boxes 2** and **3**).

These needs are expressed and may be met in families, at work and on the streets, in schools and neighbourhoods, in prisons and hospitals. Reducing structural barriers to mental health and introducing policies which protect mental well-being will benefit those who do and do not currently have mental health problems and the many people who move between periods of mental health and mental illness.

The acknowledgement that everyone has mental health needs is an important pre-condition for social inclusion, notably in the workplace. The alternative is a survival of the fittest culture, which makes a few grudging concessions to people with mental health problems, prompted mainly by fear of litigation.

It is a profound irony that many of the 'reasonable adjustments' required under the *Disability Discrimination Act* would benefit anyone who has children, relationships or elderly parents, anyone who has worries about money, alcohol, friends or housing, anyone experiencing bereavement, illness or crime. Anyone who has a life in fact.

 © THE SAINSBURY CENTRE FOR MENTAL HEALTH, 2002

BOX 2 NSF Standard One: mental health promotion

Aim

To ensure health and social services promote mental health and reduce the discrimination and social exclusion associated with mental health problems.

Health and social services should:

- promote mental health for all, working with individuals and communities;
- combat discrimination against individuals and groups with mental health problems;
- promote their social inclusion.

Meeting Standard One will require action across whole populations, as well as programmes for individuals at risk.

Performance will be assessed nationally by improvements in the psychological health of the population measured by the National Psychiatric Morbidity Survey and by a reduction in suicide rates. At a local level health improvement programmes (HImPs) should include evidence of action to:

- combat discrimination against the social exclusion of people with mental health problems;
- promote mental health in schools, workplaces and neighbourhoods; for individuals at risk and for the most vulnerable groups.

BOX 3 NSF Standard One: performance management framework by March 2002

- develop and agree an evidence-based mental health promotion strategy based on local needs assessment;
- build into local mental health promotion strategy action to promote mental health in specific settings, based on local needs;
- build into local mental health promotion strategies action to reduce discrimination;
- written care plan for those on the 'enhanced care programme approach' must show plans to secure suitable employment or other occupational activity, adequate housing and their appropriate entitlement to welfare benefits;
- implement strategy to promote employment of people with mental health problems within health and social services.

© THE SAINSBURY CENTRE FOR MENTAL HEALTH, 2002

Mental health promotion

Mental health promotion involves any action to enhance the mental well-being of individuals, families, organisations or communities.

Mental health promotion is essentially concerned with:

- how individuals, families, organisations and communities think and feel;
- the factors which influence how we think and feel, individually and collectively;
- the impact that this has on overall health and well-being.

Mental health promotion works at three levels that are relevant to the whole population; to individuals at risk; to vulnerable groups, and to people with mental health problems. In this way it works by:

- strengthening individuals – or increasing emotional resilience through interventions designed to promote self-esteem, life and coping skills, such as communicating, negotiating, relationship and parenting skills;
- strengthening communities. This involves increasing social inclusion and participation, improving neighbourhood environments, developing health and social services that support mental health, anti-bullying strategies at school, workplace health, community safety, childcare and self-help networks;
- reducing structural barriers to mental health – through initiatives to reduce racism, discrimination and inequalities and to promote access to education, meaningful employment, housing, services and support for vulnerable people.

The benefits of mental health promotion

It is often argued that mental health promotion is not relevant to people with mental health problems. This view is being challenged in the face of growing evidence of the limitations of medical models of care (see **box 4**). This means re-thinking and expanding definitions of treatment to identify what an individual needs to regain or hold onto a life that has meaning for them (Dunn, 1999; Grant, 2000; Faulkner and Layzell, 2000).

This engagement with the whole person lies at the heart of social inclusion in its true sense. It is driven by respect, reciprocity, shared decision making, an emphasis on people's strengths, a belief that everyone can make a contribution and a model of recovery, rather than illness. These values provide a framework against which the culture of the organisation and individual practice can be assessed.

 © THE SAINSBURY CENTRE FOR MENTAL HEALTH, 2002

Consultation and patient involvement are fundamental to the modernisation agenda, outlined in the NHS Plan. For local authorities, *Best Value* requires widespread consultation on services. Both will require a greater focus on quality of life indicators which impact on how people feel. Given that lack of control and lack of influence are independent risk factors for stress, how people feel about services may be as significant as clinical indicators of effectiveness (Rose, 2001). There is both an ethical and a public health case for enabling people to influence the decisions that affect their lives.

In many ways, Standard One underpins the successful delivery of the whole National Service Framework. It also provides an opportunity for those working to promote mental health **and** those delivering secondary care to work towards a shared goal of building supportive services and hospitable communities.

BOX 4 Mental health promotion can

- improve physical health and well-being;
- assist recovery from mental health problems;
- improve mental health services and the quality of life for people experiencing mental health problems;
- strengthen the capacity of communities to support social inclusion, tolerance and participation and reduce vulnerability to socio-economic stressors;
- increase the mental health literacy of individuals, organisations and communities;
- improve health at work, increasing productivity and job satisfaction.

Social inclusion in practice

It is important to recognise that social inclusion is not an intervention or a treatment (see **box 5**), but a set of values and principles that inform policy, culture, attitudes and practice. To 'deliver' social inclusion is to risk imposing another set of imperatives, which further disempower those who use services.

This means that while mental health professionals can be a catalyst for breaking down barriers, social inclusion is about landlords and tenancy agreements, job centres and benefits officers, insurance companies, employers, credit unions, timebanks, citizens advice bureaux, primary care, pubs, art galleries, adult education, leisure centres, hairdressers, neighbours and the Independent Living Fund.

BOX 5 Principles and values: empowerment and inclusion in practice

- respect
- reciprocity
- equity
- building trust
- valuing cultural diversity
- addressing race, gender and sexuality
- facilitating participation
- promoting access of information
- developing life skills
- building supporting networks
- addressing underlying feelings of powerlessness
- shared decision making

(Adapted from Dodd & Loeb, 1998)

Many frontline staff already know that addressing these wider issues improves physical and mental health, reduces the likelihood of relapse and promotes recovery. However in practice, they face major obstacles to change. Overcoming these will require a change in culture which has already begun in some mental health services (Sayce and Morris 1999). But it will also require changes in policy and practice across all sectors. The extent to which people with mental health problems are effectively denied citizenship and prevented from enjoying the same opportunities as everyone else will need to be tackled at a strategic level.

Labour MP Tony Benn is said to have asked people in positions of power:

> *"What power have you got? Where did you get it from? In whose interests do you exercise it? To whom are you accountable? How do we get rid of you?"*

We need a parallel set of questions, from the perspective of people with mental health problems, addressed to the chairs of committees, local strategic partnerships, modernisation boards, task forces, implementation teams and other bodies charged with decision making and allocation of resources at a local level.

 © THE SAINSBURY CENTRE FOR MENTAL HEALTH, 2002

Key opportunities include community strategies (www.dtlr.gov.uk), community safety partnerships (www.homeoffice.gov.uk), neighbourhood renewal (copies of the Social Exclusion Unit's *National Strategy for Neighbourhood Renewal* can be downloaded from www.cabinet-office.gov.uk/seu), regional cultural consortia (Department of Culture, Media and Sport, www.culture.gov.uk), regional development agencies (www.dtlr.gov.uk), regional chambers and regional assemblies. Other initiatives that need to ensure that a commitment to social inclusion extends to users and survivors are listed in **box 6**.

BOX 6 Related initiatives

Health:

- Health Improvement Programmes
- Health Action Zones
- Healthy Living Centres.

Education:

- Sure Start
- Education Action Zones
- Children's Fund
- Connexions
- Healthy Schools Programme
- Excellence in the Cities
- Millennium volunteering.

Employment:

- Employment Action Zones
- New Deal for Disabled People
- New Deal for Older People
- Healthy workplace initiatives.

Neighbourhoods:

- New Deal for Communities
- Regeneration
- Community strategies
- Neighbourhood renewal
- Local strategic partnerships.

These and many other initiatives can make an important contribution to the social inclusion agenda, but only if work in progress is more widely shared, with many more opportunities to debate how success is measured. There is an urgent need for resources for dissemination and evaluation, so that future investment is influenced by the priorities of those who are excluded, rather than those who, for so long, have been managing the exclusion.

© THE SAINSBURY CENTRE FOR MENTAL HEALTH, 2002

Case studies

Using mental health promotion to achieve social inclusion

The case studies below draw on different models for achieving social inclusion:

- supporting and empowering service users to access mainstream community opportunities (**case study 1**);
- changing organisational culture through user-led input (**case study 2**);
- building a strategy that combines developing alternative services, challenging mainstream service provision and addressing wider structural barriers to mental health (**case study 3**).

The projects aimed to:

- increase mental health literacy;
- build capacity and support within existing community resources;
- develop partnerships with services outside the mental health sector.

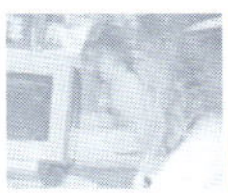

Case Study 1 Access to mainstream community opportunities

Evidence

There is growing evidence of the health and social benefits of exercise, as well as its effectiveness in reducing some symptoms, notably of depression, among people with a diagnosis. People with mental health problems are at much greater risk of physical health problems, many of which are undetected. A number of studies show that the physical health needs of people with mental health problems are neglected.

Setting

- day therapy unit (NHS);
- local gyms (privately run).

Target group

- people with mental health problems.

 © THE SAINSBURY CENTRE FOR MENTAL HEALTH, 2002

Aims

The programme aims to promote the mental health and physical fitness of people with mental health problems who access day centre facilities. It also aims to increase the confidence of local mental health service users to use non-NHS facilities within the community in which they live, and increase contact and awareness of mental health issues within the community. The programme also provides a basis for a study into the effects of exercise on people with diagnosed mental health problems, focusing on self-esteem, confidence and 'mood lifting'.

Programme

The programme is delivered by a multi-professional team including physiotherapists, occupational therapists and the day therapy team. The programme will enable clients to access community settings within a supportive environment.

Action

Two groups of ten clients with a range of diagnosed mental health problems are supported in attending a privately run gym once a week. Two members of staff from the day therapy team attend with them. The ten-week programme is monitored and evaluated with pre and post testing. Following the ten-week trial stage, clients are encouraged to continue to use the gym in a support group and it is hoped eventually independently.

Proven outcomes

- increased numbers of people with mental health problems using local community facilities;
- positive feedback from clients and staff at day centre and gym;
- positive changes in self-esteem, mood and fitness levels.

Contact

Liz Timms and Alison Luker
Avon and Western Wiltshire Mental Healthcare NHS Trust
Barrow Hospital, Barrow Gurney, Bristol BS48 3SG
Tel 0117 928 6547, Fax: 0117 928 6656
Email Alison.Luker@Awwt.swest.nhs.uk

 © THE SAINSBURY CENTRE FOR MENTAL HEALTH, 2002

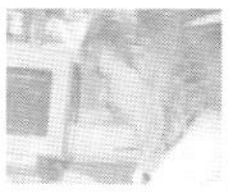

Case Study 2 User-led education – changing attitudes

Evidence

There is some evidence that interactive user-led programmes that allow young people to openly express their fears and anxieties can be effective in shifting attitudes.

Social contact with people who experience mental health problems can be a powerful solvent of prejudice and the fear and misunderstanding surrounding mental health issues.

Setting

- schools.

Target group

- whole school;
- young people at risk or vulnerable;
- young people with mental health problems.

Aims

The programme, delivered by users, aims to enable pupils and teachers of local secondary schools to increase their awareness and understanding of mental health issues and how they impact on people's lives. The programme also enables pupils and teachers to recognise the potential causes of mental ill health, signs of distress and sources of help available, locally and nationally.

Programme

The pilot project began after concern was raised in Dartford and Gravesham Mind about the unmet need for information in schools relating to stigma and mental health issues. Consultation began in local schools, which identified support for the project among teaching staff and pupils.

Action

This pilot project evaluated the effectiveness of mental health promotion literature and action in secondary schools in the local area. At the end of the pilot recommendations were made for future investment. A total of 15 sessions were held in six schools, including seven workshops on stress and stress management, two on bullying, stigma and discrimination, four on mental health awareness and two assembly sessions for all pupils on general awareness and sources of help.

 © THE SAINSBURY CENTRE FOR MENTAL HEALTH, 2002

Proven outcomes

- increased knowledge about mental health issues among pupils (78%);
- increased willingness to raise or discuss problems (66%);
- reduction of stigmatising beliefs about mental health and those who experience mental health problems (100%);
- continued work in all schools involved in the pilot to promote mental health.

Contact

Jon Manzoni
Dartford & Gravesham Mind, 16 West Hill, Dartford, Kent
Tel 01322 291380, Fax: 01322 285294.
Website www.dgmind.freeserve.co.uk
Email mail@dgmind.freeserve.co.uk

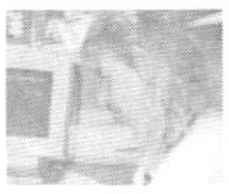

Case Study 3 Mellow – meeting the needs of young African and Caribbean men

Evidence

African and Caribbean men are over-represented in psychiatric services, and are less likely to be offered counselling or alternative therapies. Needs assessment with young African and Caribbean men with mental health problems in East London demonstrated a strong demand for services which offer a holistic approach, promote greater user involvement in decision making and recognise the impact of racism on people's experiences of everyday life.

Setting

- community and mental health services.

Target group

- young African and Caribbean men.

Aims

Mellow (men emotionally low looking for other ways) campaigns for better mental health services for young African and Caribbean men living in East London and aims to reduce psychiatric admission rates for this group. Mellow brings together those who use services, their carers, and those who work in services, as well as individuals willing to use their influence to promote the organisation. Mellow also aims to reach young men who do not engage with services and to build a programme that meets their needs.

Programme

Mellow works at a number of different levels. It runs personal development programmes for young African and Caribbean men with mental health difficulties. The 'Mellowship' programme uses arts based interventions to raise awareness of mental health issues and to enhance mental well-being among young black men.

The next development will be three resource centres that offer a holistic service, from the perspective of the social and political realities of being an African and Caribbean man in British society. The centres will offer a combination of talking therapies, outreach, employment and training opportunities. Mellow is also promoting a race and mental health forum, to build a clear strategy for tackling racism and racial inequality, without which young black men will continue to be feared and misunderstood in mental health services.

Proven outcomes

The Mellow programme is ongoing and will require long-term evaluation to assess its impact on psychiatric admissions. Interim indicators include:

- increased support for mental health issues within the African and Caribbean community;
- increased recognition, resources and strategic support for existing community and voluntary initiatives, which are often marginalised by mainstream service providers;
- success in reaching young men in the target group who do not usually access services;
- establishment of partnerships involving arts, creativity, alternative therapies, employment and training which will form the basis of a holistic approach.

Contact

Sandra Griffiths
The Mellow Campaign
East London & City Mental Health Trust
Trust Headquarters
St Clement's Hospital
2a Bow Road
London E3 4LL

Email sandra.griffiths@elcmht.nhs.uk

 © THE SAINSBURY CENTRE FOR MENTAL HEALTH, 2002

Key points

- Are you redefining what it means to be a citizen or offering rewards for conformity? Sort your activities into these categories and think about the result.
- What alliances have you formed with other 'excluded, vilified and marginalised groups'?
- Long-term mental illness is often accompanied by a variety of physical health problems. How are you (a) promoting healthy lifestyles, and (b) supporting users to obtain good primary healthcare?
- Do you know anyone who has carried out a mental health impact assessment? Locate some people who are interested in pursuing this in your community.
- What is being done to (a) strengthen individuals, (b) strengthen communities and (c) reduce structural barriers to mental health?

 © THE SAINSBURY CENTRE FOR MENTAL HEALTH, 2002

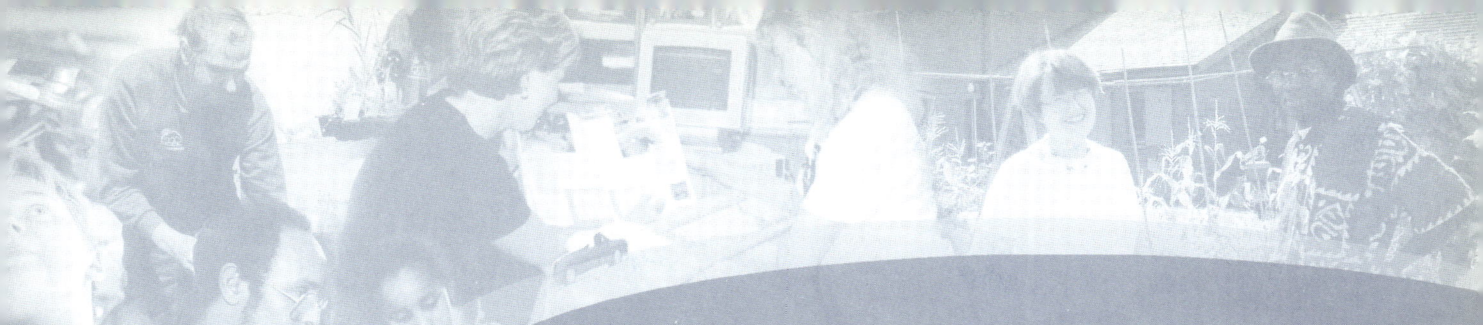

Inclusion as a new paradigm: CIVIL RIGHTS

Liz Sayce

> *"Based on seven years of work, I find that two distinct groups of persons with disabilities – those with intellectual and those with psychiatric disabilities – are systematically more marginalised and isolated than other groups of disabled people…*
>
> *"…Modern disability policy creates a motion from exclusion towards inclusion. It is high time that the most vulnerable groups amongst disabled people, including persons with psychiatric disabilities, are included in this worldwide development. To achieve this is a responsibility we must all share."*
>
> (United Nations Special Rapporteur on Disability, 2001)

Opportunities in disability rights policy

Disability rights policy, which covers those with psychiatric impairments and learning difficulties as well as sensory and physical impairments, creates significant opportunities for mental health service users. But the opportunities are not being fully grasped.

In 1990s Britain disabled people in general gained ground in terms of social inclusion, for example:

- from 1996, implementation of the first phases of the *Disability Discrimination Act 1995* (DDA), which outlaws discrimination against disabled people in employment and goods and services;
- commitment in the 1997 Labour Manifesto to 'comprehensive and enforceable civil rights for disabled people';
- the beginning of a cultural shift. In the late 1990s Glen Hoddle, manager of the England football team, was forced to resign after suggesting that disability was a punishment for sins in a past life. In 2000 paralympic athlete Tanni Grey-Thompson could not access the stage in her wheelchair to receive the award of sportswoman of the year: a mortified BBC issued an immediate prime-time apology. In 2001 Tony Blair promised to mainstream disability through all government advertising and DIY retailers B&Q deliberately profiled disabled staff in television adverts… disability became fashionable.

- passage of the *SEN (Special Educational Needs) and Disability Act 2001*, making discrimination in education on grounds of disability illegal for the first time (from September 2002);
- acceptance by government in 2001 that other loopholes in the DDA 1995 should be plugged: employees working for small companies, previously exempt, would be protected from discrimination, as would fire officers, police officers and people with HIV or cancer from the point of diagnosis.

However, inclusion of people with mental health problems remains distinctly unfashionable. Making discriminatory comments about user/survivors does not end in resignation. In 2000, tabloid newspaper, *The Sun's* editor did not resign following the headline: 'Nuts to be caged for life by docs' (*The Sun*, 2000). Companies are not vying with one another to demonstrate their corporate social responsibility by publicly employing people with mental health problems.

Indeed, a 2001 evaluation of the government's ONE programme, designed to increase employment opportunities for people excluded from the labour market, found that despite acute labour shortages only 37% of employers said they would in future take on people with mental illness. This compared to 62% who would take on physically disabled people, 78% long-term unemployed people and 88% lone parents (Department of Work and Pensions, 2001).

People with physical and sensory impairments have begun to find public support for equal rights. Mental health service users have seen the signs going the other way: increased 'not in my backyard' campaigns (Repper *et al.*, 1997), hardening public attitudes – at least until the late 1990s (Sayce, 2000) and legislative proposals focused on constraints on liberty.

The irony of this comparison is that the DDA 1995 covers people with mental health problems. By 2001 23% of all DDA employment cases were taken by people with psychiatric impairments. But this is a little known fact.

The comparison suggests that the mental health community needs to radically re-think its strategy for social inclusion. Of course the achievements in relation to disability overall have not gone far enough. But the early signs of new positive rights, achieved by disabled people's activism, give some hope for change.

Conversely, for people with severe mental health problems, rates of exclusion represent an emergency. Over the last decade the proportion who are actually working (amongst those of working age) has consistently remained below 20% – the lowest rate of any group of disabled people.

 © THE SAINSBURY CENTRE FOR MENTAL HEALTH, 2002

This could change. Those with influence in the mental health community could identify genuinely effective approaches to increasing inclusion, and then work to ensure they are agreed by stakeholders, implemented and vigorously publicised. This article is a contribution to a consideration of how to achieve the changed focus required.

Put the strategic focus for change beyond mental health services

> *"The great irony about service user action in the past 15 years is that while the position of service users within services has undoubtedly improved, the position of service users in society has deteriorated. As a result, it is at least arguable that the focus of user involvement needs adjustment."* (Peter Campbell, 2000).

History suggests that it is unwise to assume that if mental health services are first reformed wider changes will follow. The opposite strategy is much more promising: first take active steps to enable people with mental health problems to work, raise children and participate in their communities. This requires user/survivors and allies to challenge powerful forces of discrimination.

Once people with psychiatric impairments become more prominent as colleagues and fellow citizens, then a new spotlight is likely to be thrown on mental health services that are low quality or excessively coercive. Increasing user involvement and user power within services, though vital, is not enough.

Education, education – and litigation

"There is no greater problem in the field of mental health internationally than stigma." (Professor Norman Sartorius, World Psychiatric Association (WPA), 2001).

There is a growing and welcome recognition amongst mental health professionals and policy makers that challenging discrimination or stigma is top priority. (For discussions of the relative merits of the concepts 'stigma', 'discrimination' and 'social exclusion' see Sayce, 1998 and Link and Phelan, 2001. This chapter uses 'discrimination', as it better focuses attention on challenging the perpetrators. But I use 'stigma' when quoting authors who prefer that term).

The global programme to reduce stigma and discrimination in relation to schizophrenia, led by Professor Sartorius, is triggering new initiatives and research across the world. At a 2001 global conference in Leipzig, Germany, reports ranged from work on the 'Dignity of patients with schizophrenia in Islam and the Quran', targeting Egyptian Moslem leaders, to British school and media programmes (Byrne, 2000).

 © THE SAINSBURY CENTRE FOR MENTAL HEALTH, 2002

A note of caution is warranted, with respect to the effectiveness of campaigns based purely on education or imparting of knowledge.

The first pilot initiative of the WPA campaign took place in Calgary, Canada. Amongst successful strands of the campaign was an initiative to improve the way staff in an emergency room (accident and emergency) responded to people in mental health crisis.

This was not achieved by increasing knowledge or awareness amongst the staff. They already had knowledge about mental health issues, but were not (before the programme) motivated to change their practice. Instead success arose from using the persuasion of the WPA to influence the single decision-maker who could require changes (through 'regulation' of emergency rooms).

Link and Phelan, in a major review of work on stigma, point out that it depends on power. Initiatives to challenge it will therefore only succeed if they "either produce fundamental changes in attitudes and beliefs (of powerful groups) or change the power relations that underlie the ability of dominant groups to act on their attitudes and beliefs" (Link and Phelan, 2001).

Staff in the emergency room changed their behaviour because of a policy change, achieved through use of informal power – the influence of the WPA.

Sometimes informal power is not enough. Another campaign strand in Calgary was unsuccessful: the attempt to change attitudes through improved local media coverage of mental health issues. Although the team succeeded in increasing positive mental health stories by 35%, it did not bargain for an increase in negative stories of 44% for schizophrenia and 10% for mental illness (Warner, 2000). These included the story of a Canadian 'intruder' into the prime minister's residence and several high profile United States stories, including the Unibomber and the killing of two police officers at the Capitol in Washington.

Professor Arboleda-Florez (2001) of Calgary concluded that the campaign team had not given sufficient attention to potential negative outcomes. The single focus he now believed was most important was legislative change, to place controls on negative behaviours.

This conclusion comes as no surprise to British disability commentators. During the last Conservative government, one of the biggest criticisms of the *Disability Discrimination Act* was that it had no enforcement body. Instead the National Disability Council was established simply to advise and encourage good practice.

But persuasion and education, the activists contended, had no effect over several decades – a view which the Labour government accepted in 1999 when they legislated to abolish the National Disability Council in favour of the Disability Rights Commission (DRC). The DRC

 © THE SAINSBURY CENTRE FOR MENTAL HEALTH, 2002

powers include supporting individuals who wish to take cases to court or tribunal under the *Disability Discrimination Act 1995*.

Since the DRC came into being in April 2000 it has supported a number of cases concerning employment discrimination faced by people with mental health problems.

For example, Ms Marshall applied for a job as a fingerprinting officer with a police force and was offered the job – only to have the offer withdrawn when occupational health screening revealed her diagnosis of manic depression. In 2001 she won her DDA case and received nearly £20,000 in compensation. She is now working successfully elsewhere.

Also in 2001 Ms Melanophy – a successful customer services manager in an educational publishing company – challenged her employers after they sacked her for misconduct while she was a psychiatric inpatient. Her performance and conduct had been affected temporarily by a 'high' phase. The Tribunal ruled that the employer had discriminated against her and not followed its own disciplinary procedures. It is quite reasonable for an employer to expect good performance and conduct – but not to fire someone without exploring why their behaviour may have changed and what might resolve the situation. Ms Melanophy too is now working successfully elsewhere.

Sometimes the threat of the law is enough. Mr Watkiss – whose offer of a senior job with a construction company was withdrawn after his diagnosis of schizophrenia came to light – challenged the company under the DDA. The company settled, admitting unlawful discrimination and providing substantial compensation.

Cases such as these are beginning to make employers aware that they cannot discriminate with impunity; and that practical ways forward are possible. The Disability Rights Commission actively offers a velvet glove – support to achieve good practice and promotion of the major benefits of an inclusive workforce; but the employer knows there is an iron fist in the glove, which can give them extra encouragement to listen.

Initiatives that rely simply on imparting information will not motivate changes in behaviour. They need to go beyond the naïve – but still common – belief that informing people of how common mental health problems are (one in four) or increasing people's knowledge base about what mental illness is, will somehow miraculously result in reduced discrimination. There is no evidence for this belief.

Challenging discrimination effectively is a highly complex task. Sayce (2000) argues that the most promising strategy is to combine enforcement of legal rights – the iron fist – with work to change powerful beliefs in public and policy debate, coupled with practical, grassroots initiatives that change the nature of interaction between people with – and without – mental health problems.

 © THE SAINSBURY CENTRE FOR MENTAL HEALTH, 2002

Law on its own will not suffice – as the *Americans with Disabilities Act* shows, without sufficient promotion and real understanding of the benefits of an inclusive society. The powers of this Act have been pared back through judicial and political interpretation. But nor is education sufficient on its own, as Arboleda-Florez makes clear. To paraphrase Link and Phelan (2001), we need **both** to change the attitudes and beliefs of those with power **and** to place real constraints on the use of that power, for example through legal sanctions.

Initiatives to tackle discrimination must also be led by user/survivors, so the work itself models the shift in power that is sought. There is overwhelming evidence that attitudes are far more likely to be changed through education by people with mental health problems than other 'educators' (Sayce, 2000; Warner, 2000).

The law is not the only way to tackle power; using influence or the power of embarrassment can be enough. For instance in the US concerted lobbying has led to withdrawal of discriminatory advertisements and soap opera lines. Superman would have been killed by an escapee from an inter-galactic asylum, were it not for the efforts of mental health campaigners (Wahl, 1995).

Disability rights – not illness rights

When ex-president Clinton grasped the concept of 'psychiatric disability' he translated it into action for civil rights at the heart of the federal government:

> *"One of our goals is to help people understand that mental illness is not a character flaw. It is a disability... That is why today I am using my executive authority to strip away outdated barriers that keep people with psychiatric disabilities from serving America in our federal government."*
> Bill Clinton (remarks at the US Disability Awards Ceremony, June 1999)

The term 'disability' focuses attention on the relationship between the individual and the society which discriminates. Under the social model of disability a person is disabled not – or not just – by their impairment (being blind, or unable to walk, or having difficulties in thinking or feeling) but by the barriers that society puts in their way. The disability movement therefore focuses its efforts on pulling down the barriers – which may be attitudinal, structural, economic or physical – to enable people to participate.

The individual with a psychiatric impairment, by contrast, is a 'patient', a 'client', a 'user', a 'consumer' or a 'survivor' of **the services**. This entrenches the idea that the key relationship is between the individual and mental health services – and that to improve matters, changes

© THE SAINSBURY CENTRE FOR MENTAL HEALTH, 2002

in the services are needed. This is just the limited vision that Peter Campbell critiques. If, by contrast, the individual is a disabled person, someone with a psychiatric impairment, the focus goes back where it belongs, on the relationship with society as a whole.

There are other reasons for the mental health community to join – and add its distinctive voice to – the wider disability movement and its allies.

'Illness' is not a useful concept to describe the experience of people with long-term mental health problems. Illness suggests an episode, during which the person needs to be relieved of responsibilities, as employee or parent, until they 'get better'. Disability is something you live with; it does not prevent you from having responsibilities, given support as necessary and removal of external barriers. The disabled person can normally work or continue parenting whether they 'get better' or not. Hope is not contingent on cure, but on 'recovery' in the sense of finding meaning and fulfilment with the impairment.

Evidence suggests that when the public understands the message that 'mental illness is an illness like any other', which underpins so many anti-stigma campaigns across the world, they become more likely to believe the person is incapable and not responsible: a poor unfortunate, rather than an equal citizen. As Read and Harre put it, the mental illness/brain disease messages are related to:

> *"Negative attitudes, including perceptions that 'mental patients' are dangerous, anti-social and unpredictable, with reluctance to become romantically involved with them.*
>
> *"... It is recommended that destigmatisation programmes consider abandoning efforts to promulgate illness-based explanations and focus instead on increasing contact with and exposure to users of mental health services."* (Read and Harre, 2001).

Given the need to tackle the power that fuels discrimination it makes no sense to start with a concept like 'brain disease', which evokes images of powerlessness. Current German anti-stigma campaigns based on concepts such as 'Crazy – so what?' and 'Normal to be different' are far more promising (Angermeyer, 2001).

Employers respond very negatively to the 'illness' concept. 'Ill' people should not be at work, almost by definition. They should be tucked up in bed. If they are employed, it is assumed (wrongly in this case) that they are likely to have a great deal of sick leave and be a bad employment risk. But employers are beginning to understand that disabled people can and do work – and may need 'reasonable adjustments' in order to do so (for instance, being able to call a friend or mental health worker from work during difficult times).

 © THE SAINSBURY CENTRE FOR MENTAL HEALTH, 2002

Approaching employers with the message that they may like to employ 'mentally ill people' is a recipe for disaster. Suggesting they take on disabled people is a very different matter. Supported employment programmes based on a disability model also appear to have greater success than those based on an illness model: illness models are premised on short-term progress into unsupported work. Whereas disability models can offer fluctuating, longer term support as needed (Secker *et al.*, 2001).

The DDA 1995 is the only law in the last decade to have increased rights for people with mental health problems. When 23% of employment cases under this law concern people with psychiatric impairments, it would be neglectful, based on the evidence, not to draw on this source of power, to underpin social inclusion strategies. It can act as the effective iron fist behind the velvet glove of educational and practical approaches.

Key points

The achievement of social inclusion requires:

- leadership of initiatives by user/survivors. If power is to shift, user/survivors need to lead the moves for change, with mental health professionals and others playing an invaluable role as allies;
- a focus beyond mental health services – on wider issues of power and rights;
- effective use of tools to address abuses of power: particularly the legal protections of disability discrimination laws, as a vital backdrop to educational and practical initiatives;
- use of a disability, not an illness, conceptualisation: disabled people can make powerful contributions, where people with illnesses of the brain are seen as incompetent.

Finally, international links are vital. As the UN Rapporteur notes, the policy shift towards social inclusion of all disabled people is international. The benefits need to be realised for some of the most excluded disabled people of all – those with psychiatric impairments.

© THE SAINSBURY CENTRE FOR MENTAL HEALTH, 2002

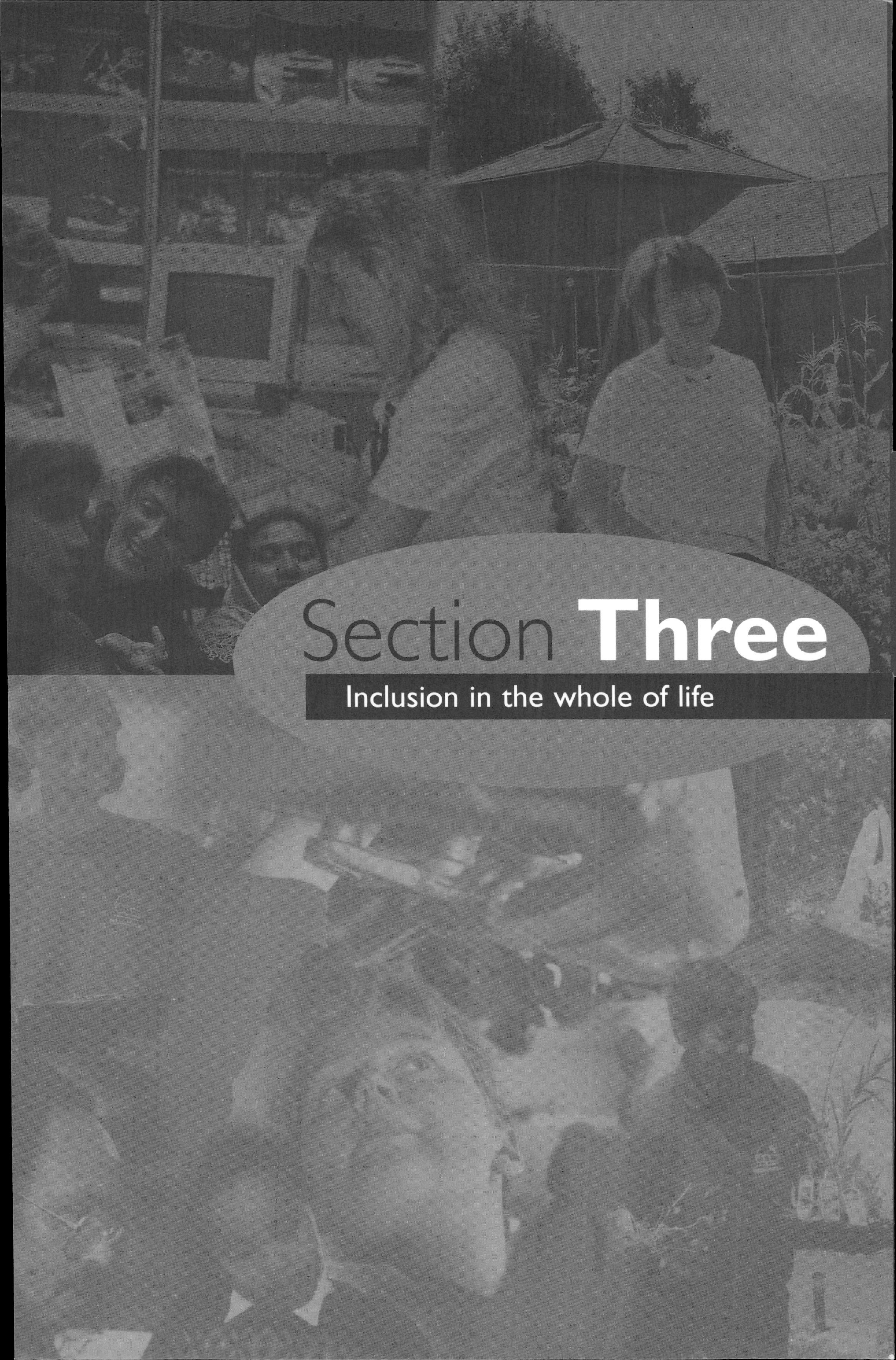

Section **Three**

Inclusion in the whole of life

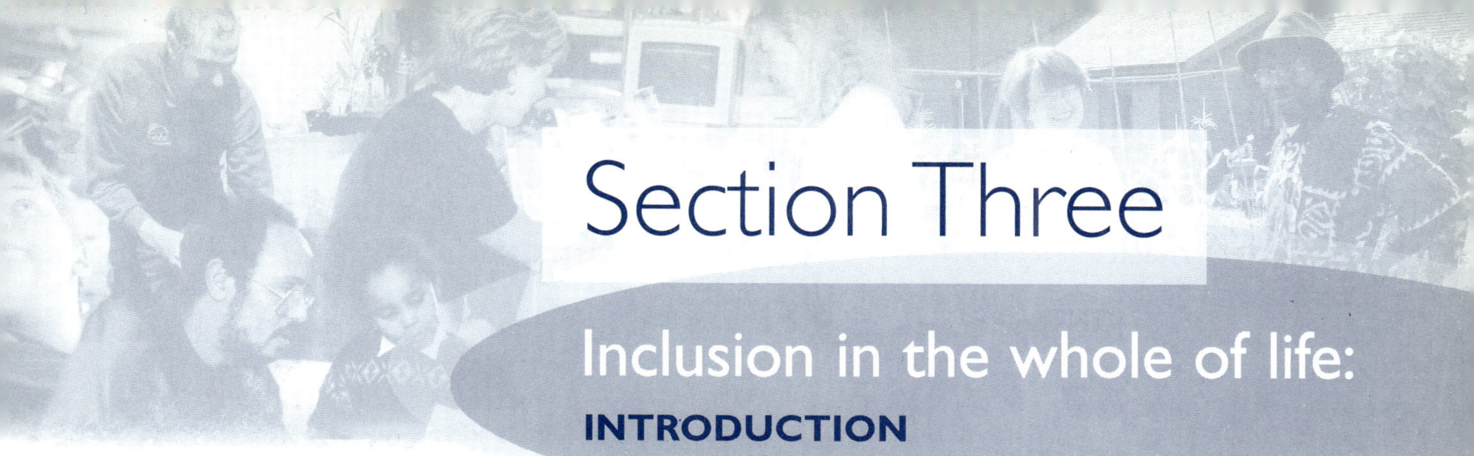

Section Three

Inclusion in the whole of life: INTRODUCTION

Peter Bates

So far this resource book has focused upon some of the key ideas and approaches that have formed the basis for an inclusive approach to mental health. In this section we look at a number of specific projects that illustrate how people with mental health difficulties engage in the whole of life.

In *Growing Strong Communities*, David Boyle and Zoe Reed give a description of community timebanks in the United States and the United Kingdom. These new organisations bring local citizens together to contribute their skills and abilities to each other and to the community as a whole. People shift from receiving healthcare to contributing, from a focus on their problems to their abilities, from vertical relationships with professionals to horizontal relationships with their neighbours. Dependency is replaced by reciprocity in the shared goal of growing strong communities.

These community timebanks encourage people to give and receive time. There is also a separate national media campaign called timebank that encourages people to pledge their time as volunteers in their local community. The networking organisation for community timebanks can be found at www.timebanks.co.uk while the media campaign is at www.timebank.org.uk.

While community timebanks provide a vibrant illustration of the principle of reciprocity, there have been other initiatives that have similar objectives. Local exchange trading schemes (LETS), credit unions, healthy living centres and GP referral schemes can all bring people with mental health problems into closer relationships with other members of the community. Art exhibitions, poetry recitations and theatre performances take talented service users into direct and positive contact with their neighbours – into settings where talent can be appreciated and respect earned.

Vanessa Pinfold and colleagues in Kent describe an initiative that addresses issues of *Community Safety*. Many service users report that the experience of forced removal from a public place to a so-called place of safety under section 136 of the *Mental Health Act 1983* is both degrading and distressing for people in crisis. Service users identified the police as

 © THE SAINSBURY CENTRE FOR MENTAL HEALTH, 2002

one of a series of targets for mental health awareness training. The user group then went on to design, deliver and evaluate their training programme.

There are three particular elements of this work that deserve to be transferred to other programmes. First, is the way in which the service users became direct experience trainers – using their own hard-won first hand knowledge as a tool within the training programme. Moreover, service users did not merely deliver a syllabus designed elsewhere – they were involved in the programme from conception to write-up.

Second is the rigorous approach to evaluation. The team did not rely on guesswork to design the syllabus, but surveyed the perceived needs of the audience. They did not hope for a few words of thanks at the close of the event, but instead used a follow-up questionnaire to survey for attitude change. Third, the programme has begun with the police but the team plan to move on to welfare benefits staff, schools and one day, GPs.

From an inclusion perspective, there are potential audiences amongst employers, volunteer involving organisations, college tutors, librarians, lifeguards at the sports centre and so on. A similar format to the Kent approach could be applied in any other area of community life.

In the next article, Maurice Harker reflects on the history of housing services and government policy. The last decade has seen a steady move from group to individual opportunities along with a wider array of options and more individualised funding. One version of fully individualised support is called supported living (Kinsella, 1995) and comprises the following five components:

1. **Separate housing and support.** The agency that provides or co-ordinates support is not the landlord, nor does it have any organisational connection to the property owner.
2. **Focusing on one person at a time.** A process of person-centred planning is used to find out what each individual person wants, and then to plan individually and assist them in securing the accommodation and level of support that is right for them.
3. **Full user choice and control.** Individuals choose where they live, who they live with (if anyone), who supports them and how. Individuals hold their own tenancy or mortgage and are in control of their own money and household.
4. **Rejecting no one.** There is an implicit assumption that everyone can live in the community. The fact that someone has complex needs does not mean they should be denied the opportunity to choose their own lifestyle. Attention is given to environmental adaptations and individually designed supports.
5. **Focusing on relationships.** This involves making use of informal supports and community resources. The starting point is to build on a person's existing relationships and connections. Paid help is only used when natural supports are not available. Paid supporters work to develop a person's social network, alongside other activities.

 © THE SAINSBURY CENTRE FOR MENTAL HEALTH, 2002

Despite the general broadening of options, gaps remain in the availability of support for people with intensive and multiple needs, those in crisis and people seeking active skills development. Continuing to shift away from traditional housing services to models that approximate supported living remains a co-ordination challenge for those who provide housing, health and social care.

While a decent place to live is fundamental to an included lifestyle, it is sometimes the softer, cultural things that make people feel that they belong. In *The Information Age*, Melba Wilson tells the story of the cyber café run by Mind.

After the powerful inquiry report *Creating Accepting Communities* published by Mind (Dunn, 1999), a local project began to offer computer skills to people with mental health problems. Participants benefit in the fields of education, leisure and employment as well as developing confidence and a sense of connection to contemporary society.

This report also develops the theme of inter-agency partnership raised earlier by Fabian Davis and colleagues by showing how four disparate agencies came together to identify their own contributions, outcomes and to find common ground. Again, this provides a pattern for inter-agency work in a range of other fields.

The Mind project created an inclusive opportunity as a new project in the space between a number of existing organisations. In the article on *Education*, Kathryn James and Jacqueline Henderson offer a range of ideas about how further and community education providers can be more welcoming to students with mental health difficulties. They are at pains to show that this is a reciprocal arrangement, and mental health services may have some things to learn about education too.

Empowerment and participation of mental health service users is translated into participation in the college, with courses becoming more democratic, student-centred and flexible. James and Henderson present some very practical suggestions about how to support students in their learning, and how to support the college in its provision of education.

The final area opens with a review by Justine Schneider of employment initiatives for people with mental health problems. The five most common models – sheltered workshops, the transitional employment programme, social firms, vocational rehabilitation, and individual placement and support – are compared and contrasted by reference to the research literature. Employment projects provide a substantial element of mental health day opportunities in many areas, and this theme has been further stimulated by the government's Welfare to Work programme, so it is important that resources are invested in effective models.

Pentreath Industries Ltd provides an illustration of a mental health employment service that has provided a wide variety of the models reviewed by Schneider and also links with local education providers. Judgements about the appropriate models to adopt must also be taken with reference to local circumstances.

 © THE SAINSBURY CENTRE FOR MENTAL HEALTH, 2002

This section has been able to cover only a few of the potential areas of community life that might be addressed. A few additional areas are listed below, along with references to pursue further study.

- **arts** – Health Education Authority (1998)
- **faith communities** – Mental Health Foundation (2000)
- **museums** – Dodd and Sandell (2001)
- **neighbouring** – Wolff *et al.* (1996)
- **sports and exercise** – Morgan (1997)
- **voluntary work** – Bates (2002, forthcoming)

 © THE SAINSBURY CENTRE FOR MENTAL HEALTH, 2002

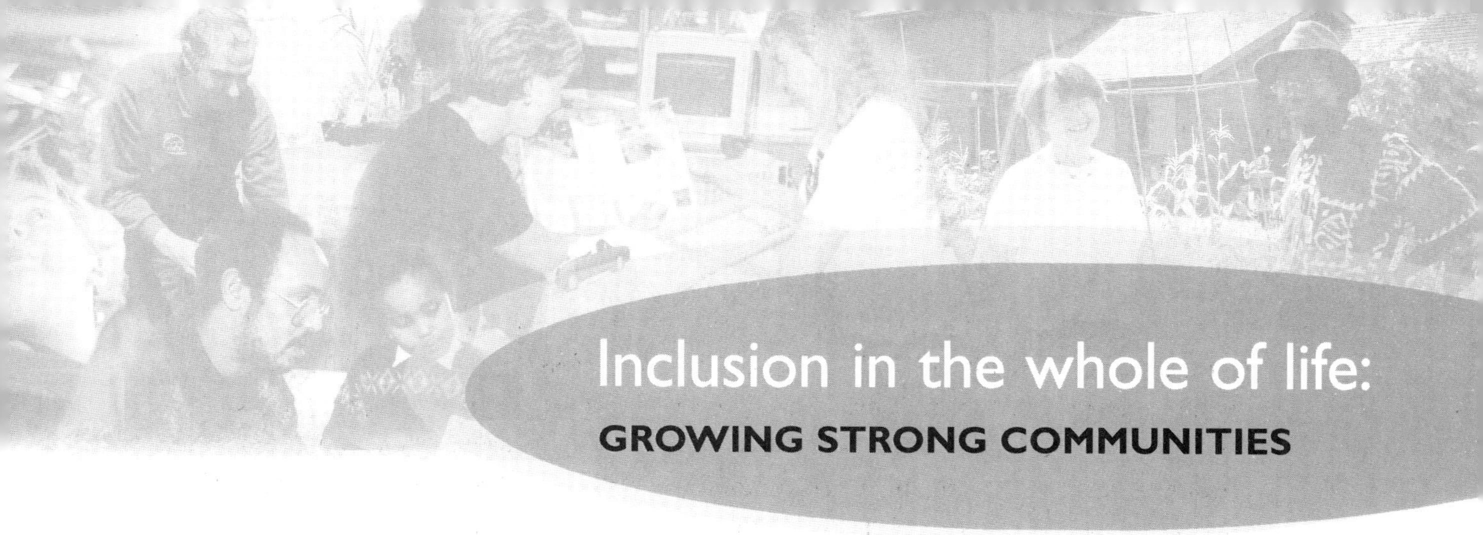

Inclusion in the whole of life:
GROWING STRONG COMMUNITIES

David Boyle and Zoe Reed

David Boyle of the New Economics Foundation writes:

It has become a truism in community development circles that professionals cannot succeed unless they enlist the equal involvement of their clients. No housing advisor, debt counsellor, or planner is going to do their job properly without doing so. They may fully succeed only rarely and the official conception of participation may be woefully inadequate, but the idea is still true.

Those working on the cusp of medicine and community – especially in mental health – are increasingly experimenting with the same thought. It isn't anything very new, after all. Everybody knows that doctors need the enthusiastic involvement of their patients to enable recovery. But what if the medical relationship became explicitly more two-way: instead of doctors delivering health to the community, maybe there is scope for this to become a more reciprocal relationship.

It is important to set out first what that relationship would not be. It would not mean that patients would pay for their treatment. On the other hand, it might mean that doctors or mental health professionals might ask for something back in terms of people's time. That is the thinking behind the idea of community timebanks, which arrived in the UK from the USA in 1998. There are now getting on for 40 of them around the country, allowing people to earn 'time credits' for the effort they put in around their local community – anything from visiting to tutoring – and to spend them when they need help themselves.

Timebanks have received the enthusiastic backing of the Government. Ministers have exempted time credits for tax and benefits, and the model has been growing fast – especially in community centres and especially for older people – just as it has been growing in Japan and China as a way of providing non-medical support to the burgeoning elderly populations. Timebanks like Fair Shares in Gloucestershire or the HourBank in Peckham have been rebuilding community networks by re-creating reciprocal relationships between people at local level.

 © THE SAINSBURY CENTRE FOR MENTAL HEALTH, 2002

But in the USA, timebanks using a currency they call 'time dollars' are becoming more specialised, revolutionising the relationships between professional and client in education, penal institutions and mental health. Teenage jurors in Washington or teenage peer tutors in Chicago are cashing in their time credits or time dollars for refurbished computers. Prisoners are earning them for keeping in touch with their children. People with depression are earning them by looking after local older people.

Running through the whole project is the central idea that it is the service users who hold the key to producing successful public services – in anything from housing to health. Take, for example, the New Economics Foundation's timebank (funded by the King's Fund) at the Rushey Green Central Clinic in Lewisham, South East London. GP Richard Byng and his team decided to experiment with the timebank approach because they wanted to get away from prescribing for problems they knew were social rather than medical in origin. They knew that, in a community with large African-Caribbean, Turkish and refugee populations – where a third of their 6,000-strong catchment changes every year – much of their patients' ill health and anxiety arose from feelings of social isolation. Many did not know where to go for help, did not know their neighbours or were too frightened to go out. Many of the families supported by the primary care team were desperately in need of simple practical support.

The timebank allowed patients to provide support and help for each other. Ultimately, where it made sense, the GPs would be able to prescribe a friendly face or a lift to the shops once a week, instead of medication. Timebank members would be encouraged to 'earn' credits by contributing skills and energies in a whole variety of ways.

The timebank was launched in March 2000 and now has more than 60 active participants, regularly visiting, dog-walking, baby-sitting, or doing anything from writing poetry to accompanying blind people shopping. Doctors are already referring patients to the bank, especially in cases of long-term depression – because they find that participation in the timebank can lead to real improvements in mental health.

Thanks to support from the Lloyds–TSB Foundation, the timebank is planning to launch a DIY team. That means volunteers will be earning 'credits' by carrying out small repairs at people's homes – anything from changing a light bulb to fitting a safety rail (one of the main factors that keep older people in hospital when they could otherwise go home after a fall). On every visit, they will also check smoke alarms and fit new ones where needed.

There are a number of immediate implications arising from this changed relationship, and not all of them sit easily within a traditional view of professional medicine:

- It makes the fact that doctors need patients as much as patients need doctors absolutely explicit. When patients are partners in the business of keeping the neighbourhood healthy, they are equals.

© THE SAINSBURY CENTRE FOR MENTAL HEALTH, 2002

- The focus shifts from people's problems to their abilities. Professionals traditionally concentrate on what patients **can't** do: often this becomes the accepted way of triggering help. Timebanks in a mental health context focus instead on people's assets, what they **can** do – and this can be an empowering experience for them. Feeling useful can be a basic human need, and anecdotal experience in Rushey Green shows that this can make a real difference to people with long-term depression.
- By using these hidden resources in the community, surgeries are able to provide access to a much wider range of services than traditional surgeries. Member to Member in Brooklyn, one of the first timebanks in the USA, allows its parent company Elderplan to advertise across New York with a picture of a timebank member of the DIY team bearing the slogan 'Does your health insurance company give you a friend like George?'

Member to Member has expanded to provide a range of self-help workshops for participants, on anything from arthritis to bereavement. Rushey Green, which has made depression a special focus, provides services like phone befriending, making and sharing meals, swimming and walking groups – anything that people can enjoy sharing together, as well as the more predictable services like baby-sitting or shopping. The King's Fund and Guy's Hospital Trustees are launching a two-year research programme on the health effects of the Rushey Green timebank, but doctors are already reporting real improvements among some of those taking part.

Experience of one timebank programme in Miami shows that it can be a place where informal care by volunteers can make a major difference in mental health. Abriendo Puertas is in East Little Havana, a high-crime, high-density and low-income neighbourhood in the racially divided city. Its central purpose is to support children and families, so that they can stay together and thrive in local schools.

Its new family centre opened in 1995 with the help of the Annie E. Casey Foundation and public funders, and has been looking for innovative ways of delivering services in a way that can cross the difficult barriers between neighbourhoods, races and ages. As a result, all participants registered in their programme agree to earn time dollars to support their activities – a reciprocal system which immediately breaks down the stigma which is sometimes associated with 'free' services and which can often get in the way of fostering mental health.

The programme has been successful enough to expand out of the family centre and provide volunteer help to other local organisations including Charlee, the local foster care programme that donates furniture and clothing to people in East Little Havana, and the Kiwanis, a local social service organisation. The result is a connected series of services, linked by time credits, which support each other. They also include:

 © THE SAINSBURY CENTRE FOR MENTAL HEALTH, 2002

- The Family Council (members of which have to earn at least five hours a month) made up of parents, custodial grandparents and foster parents of children, and which has a wide brief to organise public events and link together local schools, childcare and youth organisations.
- A system of service delivery called EQUIPO that links formal and informal care to identify, assess and meet need.
- A youth group.
- Shared Services Network, funded by the Department of Education to link parents with the Riverside Elementary School.

The services include a wide range of training, outreach, advocacy, legal advice, childcare, tutoring, and birthday celebrations – all of which are free in dollars but some of which charge in time credits. Much of the activity carried out by the 3,700 registered participants involves referring people in difficulty to the right agency before their problems become unmanageable.

Abriendo Puertas and Rushey Green are two models of timebanks that inject some reciprocity into mental health services. The timebanks themselves require little more than TimeKeeper software and someone on the end of a phone. The reciprocity can be injected (as in Miami) by charging in time for services that used to be free and unappreciated as a result. Or it can be (as in Lewisham) simply by asking patients for something back.

Both of these are a new departure in medicine. Both would deserve to be controversial if they were pushed to the limit, insisting that vulnerable patients 'pay back' in some way. But by experimenting with the idea where appropriate, both are able to make a difference to patients' lives, turning people's needs into assets and capabilities that can enrich them and others.

On the other hand, sticking too rigidly to a professionalism that allows no partnership with patients – which refuses to ask people for anything at all – can sometimes give the impression that patients have nothing of value that anybody could possibly need. The timebanks idea says that this attitude is disempowering to patients and ignores a vital new resource that can heal them and the neighbourhoods where they live.

Zoe Reed responds:

It is self evident that mental health services are struggling to cope with a tidal wave of needs and expectations. Successive governments have introduced sweeping changes in the belief that they have the right solutions for the perceived failure of health service delivery. Staff responses range from the stoic, "we can cope with anything", to the stressed and

 © THE SAINSBURY CENTRE FOR MENTAL HEALTH, 2002

distressed that are increasingly upset that the service they provide fails to meet their own high expectations. The public has been encouraged to blame the services for all society's ills and recipients of the services call themselves survivors – lucky to have escaped a brutalising system.

So maybe it is the paradigm that is wrong. Perhaps our way of thinking is blocking us from tapping a vast reservoir of resources – i.e. service users and the local communities in which they live – who could be working with us to alleviate mental distress. Perhaps the organisational learning and staff development which is required for mental health services needs to shift from the 'professional expert' mindset.

Professional experts help and do things to certain people who fit particular categories when they are ill. We propose a new model which focuses on building capacity rather than developing dependency and which works alongside people and communities wherever it suits them, to minimise the experience of mental distress everywhere and at all times.

What would the work of professionals look like if they viewed their job as working with people to achieve **their** personal and community objectives? It starts to unpack the whole notion of 'professional' – the idea that some people know what's best for people in need who come to them for help.

It shifts the focus to one of understanding that no service is a quality service unless the people who use it are treated and feel like co-producers in that service. We are not talking about a bit of customer care training here – but a fundamental paradigm shift in the way we view citizens and service users and, equally importantly, in the way we view ourselves and the contribution our professional roles make in society.

A common complaint from service users is that nurses won't talk to them. Another is that psychiatrists are arrogant and abrupt. Reciprocity thinking leads us to question the claim that we are providing a quality service, when service users feel disempowered and disengaged. Service user involvement strategies also benefit from the reciprocity perspective. If we are to involve service users in meaningful ways in the structures and processes of the organisation, then it should build upon service users feeling involved in their own care. The feeling of involvement comes from a sense that you are engaging in a real dialogue.

Dialogue is a special kind of conversation. Arthur Battram (1997), in his book *Navigating Complexity*, describes it as being about emergence – the bringing forth of new and previously hidden meanings and understandings. To successfully hold this special kind of conversation a number of rules need to be observed. One of these is 'treat everyone's views as equally valid'. Successful involvement, then, at all levels, brings you back to the concept of reciprocity.

 © THE SAINSBURY CENTRE FOR MENTAL HEALTH, 2002

This sort of thinking has prompted a number of streams of activity across our NHS Trust (South London and Maudsley) – with the promise of more to come. The board, together with Lewisham Council and the New Economics Foundation have funded a two-year part-time development worker to help timebanks grow – both within the trust and across the geographic area where we provide services (primarily Lambeth, Southwark, Lewisham and Croydon).

Timebanks generate social energy – the willingness and ability of people to act in the common interest – by developing skills, confidence, trust and shared values. They are based on the core values of:

- can do – everyone has something of value to give and we need their contribution;
- equality – everyone's time is worth the same;
- reciprocity – everyone is a giver and a receiver.

The intention is to use the timebank as a tool to build local community capacity so that people with serious, long term, mental illness can still feel they have value and worth and are able to make a contribution that is recognised and rewarded.

The timebank is a mechanism that has at its heart the notion of reciprocity. It is a way in which recognition and reward can be given to every participant. It encourages each person to both give and receive. It breaks away from the notion that some of us have things to give and others can only receive.

Currently, the following services are being reconfigured or developed to incorporate the timebank mechanism and the principles of reciprocity:

- The traditional volunteers' service attached to the Bethlem and Maudsley Hospital is being restructured to become 'mutual volunteering'. This immediately changes the nature of the relationship – emphasising that everyone gives and receives – not necessarily within the same relationship but as players within a broader community that we are building together.

  Contact: Jane.Masters@slam-tr.nhs.uk or Su.Glazier@slam-tr.nhs.uk.

- The Cares of Life Project is a major initiative currently under development that is aimed at fundamentally improving the mental health service provision for African and African Caribbean people in the Borough of Southwark. This model of service provision will harness the resources of the statutory services, the black majority churches, black voluntary organisations and the Southwark consortium of timebanks. A network of lay health workers and link workers will be deployed to use interventions, which have been developed jointly with service users, for common mental disorders that are described as

 © THE SAINSBURY CENTRE FOR MENTAL HEALTH, 2002

'cares of life' by the local black population. The project will facilitate the sharing of knowledge and skills in a reciprocal way as well as build the capacity of the local community *and* the local mental health services so that together, they can better meet the needs of black people experiencing the 'cares of life'.

Contact: Dele.Olajide@slam-tr.nhs.uk.

- In Croydon, a timebank partnership is being developed between a trust day service, two voluntary organisations and a social services day centre. All the organisations involved work with individuals who experience enduring mental health problems and who often face exclusion from ordinary social roles and situations because of this. The timebank offers a variety of opportunities for service users and staff to make equal contributions to the local community and the reciprocity goes some way to addressing the 'them and us' culture, which so often pervades service provision.

  Contact: Pam.Filson@slam-tr.nhs.uk.

- The Addictions Division is very keen to develop a timebank for its service users. It feels that substance-misusing clients, particularly those who use illicit substances, are one of the most marginalised groups in society. In general, the self-esteem of these clients is low despite being an able group. Using timebanks as a way of helping people rebuild their self-esteem will add to their quality of life as well as improve treatment outcomes.

  Contact: Claire.Parry@slam.nhs.uk.

This outward looking approach, with secondary mental health services seeing themselves as a small core supporting and sustaining local people in accessing the full range of social, economic, environmental and health services and opportunities – requires the paradigm shift in thinking which reciprocity is all about. It requires us to view each person as having resources and abilities to give to their community and to give to themselves – our role is to work alongside them so that each person can use their capacity to its maximum.

South London and Maudsley NHS Trust and New Economics Foundation are working collaboratively with a growing network of statutory, voluntary and community organisations on this mental health aspect of the London timebanks initiative. Get in touch if you want to hear how it's going or to develop the ideas in your area (see the list of contributors on p265).

 © THE SAINSBURY CENTRE FOR MENTAL HEALTH, 2002

Key points

In South London:

- Easy ways are being developed for mental health service users to 'give something back' and feel useful in their locality.
- The local council and the mental health trust have funded a worker to develop timebanks for both users and non-users of mental health services.
- Black people are redefining mental distress and designing interventions to meet their needs.
- People with mental health problems are making valued, voluntary contributions to their neighbourhood and improving their own quality of life at the same time.

 © THE SAINSBURY CENTRE FOR MENTAL HEALTH, 2002

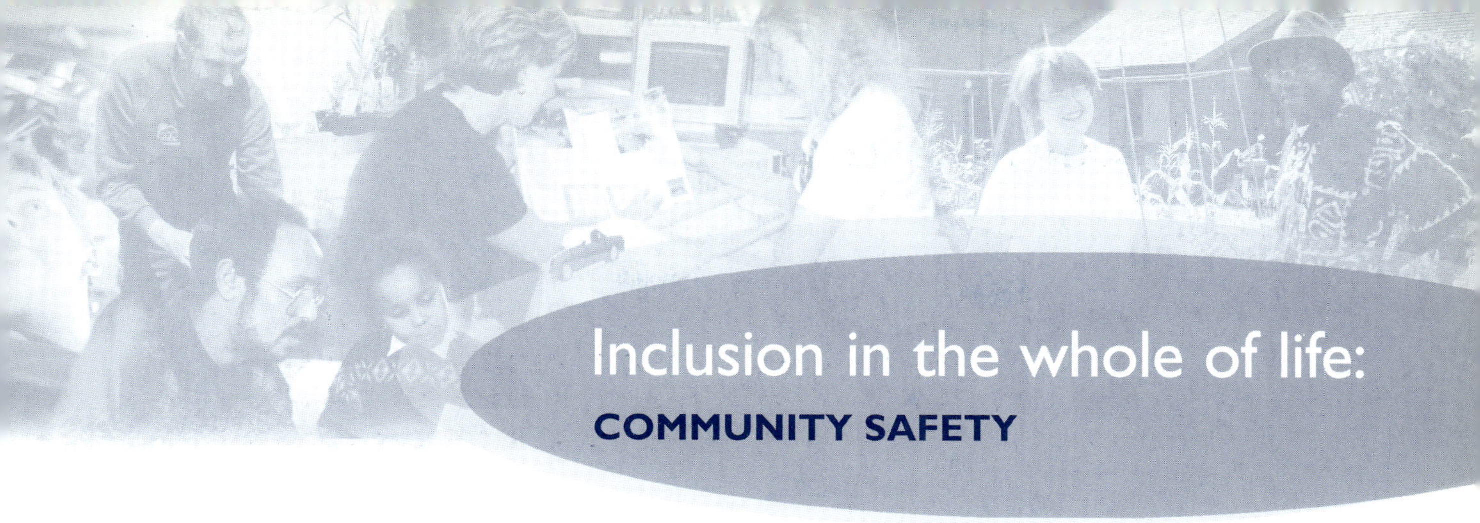

Inclusion in the whole of life:

COMMUNITY SAFETY

Vanessa Pinfold and
Kent service users

The Institute of Psychiatry, in collaboration with voluntary organisations, statutory services, service user forums and carer support groups, has been developing a programme of mental health awareness workshops for community audiences in Kent called the Kent Awareness in Action Programme. The aim is to address the stigma and discrimination experienced by people with mental health problems through mental health promotion initiatives that seek to:

- educate – provide factual information about mental illness;
- raise awareness – emphasise the importance of mental health for all;
- explore our attitudes and behaviour towards people with mental health problems.

The workshops adopt an experiential approach to discussing health and illness. Sessions are based around presentations from service users providing personal accounts of living with mental illness and discussions with the target audience about their own experiences of working with people whom they recognise to be experiencing mental distress.

This approach ensures that the workshops promote contact with people who have mental health problems, a factor shown to be important when influencing public attitudes (Angermeyer and Matschinger, 1996) and address the difficulties of changing public attitudes with information alone (Penn *et al.*, 1994). It does this by using a combination of focused learning strategies that encourages emotional participation and participant interaction in a target audience. It does not, however, tackle other aspects of the stigma process such as structural discrimination, self-stigmatisation or the cultural context of deeply held attitudes and beliefs.

Stigma, discrimination and social exclusion

The stigma of mental illness, and the discrimination and social exclusion that people with mental health problems experience, is well documented (Dunn, 1999). Stigma inhibits recovery; stops people seeking and accepting help and reduces life opportunities. Once

 © THE SAINSBURY CENTRE FOR MENTAL HEALTH, 2002

labelled with a mental illness it can be difficult to maintain or regain employment (Huxley and Thornicroft, 2000). Employers do discriminate both overtly and covertly against the stereotypes that people with mental health problems are: unpredictable, dangerous, difficult to communicate with, different, have only themselves to blame, never recover (Crisp *et al.*, 2000).

Re-building one's life after a period of illness not only involves living with any lasting effects and the side effects of medication and other treatment options, but it also involves learning to cope with public attitudes and reactions towards mental illness. People report that they are treated differently when their mental illness 'label' is disclosed (Read and Baker, 1996; Mental Heath Foundation, 2000b): kids throw a brick through your window; neighbours don't talk to you any more; the GP doesn't take your physical health problems seriously. Mental health stigma prevents people from getting involved in community activities.

Language is important for providing a frame of reference, and it is particularly important in the field of mental health. There are many contested terms for describing the mental health/mental illness continuum within the discipline and a large vocabulary of stigmatising expressions adopted by the general public and embedded in popular culture such as: 'fruit cake' 'crackers',' schizo', 'psycho', 'retard', and 'nutter'.

The Department of Health's 'Mind Out for Mental Health' campaign 2001 works with school children and targets language in its programme to reduce stigma and discrimination, in an attempt to change the way young people view and talk about mental illness.

For those working in the field of mental health the medicalisation of illness has been challenged by approaches which focus upon an everyday language describing varying levels of emotional well-being and distress, and support the continuing search for a description to replace the patient label.

In this article, we have used several terms interdependently (mental illness, mental distress, mental health problems) reflecting Kent Awareness in Action's use of both medical terminology (schizophrenia, manic depression, dual diagnosis) and a normalising approach to mental health awareness training. This approach seeks to provide the community audience with a sensitive language to discuss mental health issues whilst exploring the facts behind medical terms that they come across in the course of their work.

The social inclusion and citizenship agenda is an empowering movement that recognises and values the contributions that we can all provide in society. In policy terms the concept of social inclusion and mental health is important because it places the specific issue of stigma and discrimination against people with mental health problems within the *National Service Framework for Mental Health* (Department of Health, 1999b). This gives health and social service departments responsibilities for developing strategies to address both mental health promotion and issues related to social exclusion in the community.

 © THE SAINSBURY CENTRE FOR MENTAL HEALTH, 2002

When assessing barriers to wider participation in the local community and communities of interest for people with mental health problems, one factor to emerge is the absence of the capacity to 'care' within the community: the 'not in my backyard' public attitude that health and social care planners are initially faced with on attempting to locate facilities for people with mental health problems (Repper *et al.*, 1997).

There are of course numerous mental health system and person-specific issues that need to be addressed when promoting social inclusion. These include:

- the continued development of community mental health services;
- improved psychiatric drug treatments with fewer side effects;
- problems related to self-stigmatisation;
- improving the self-confidence and self-esteem of people who feel devalued through their illness experiences.

However, all these initiatives must be run in conjunction with programmes that help individuals and groups in the community to become more accepting of difference.

A persistent lack of education on issues relating to mental health problems leaves many in society largely ignorant and fearful of mental illness. Programmes to support and empower service users to engage in ordinary everyday activities in community, for example: return to the workplace; taking up voluntary placements; joining the sports club; attending adult education classes, will be more successful if host communities are empowered with knowledge and understanding surrounding the myths and facts of mental illness.

It may be that individuals will educate themselves, as many service users do on a daily basis. But mental health awareness projects with groups whose work brings them into contact with people with mental health problems may also go some way towards reducing stigma and discrimination by dispelling myths, challenging stereotypes, offering standards for good practice and promoting positive mental health for all:

> *"At the end of the mental health awareness project I hope that we will have achieved a sense of what it means to be aware of mental health. How people can recover given the chance to improve their lives. How being part of the project shows others what people suffering mental illness are able to do, if given the opportunity."*
> (Clifford Hayes, member of Kent Awareness in Action).

Developing mental health awareness workshops for Kent police

"Who should we target with mental health awareness interventions?" was the question posed to members of mental health forums across Kent at the beginning of the project in September 2000.

 © THE SAINSBURY CENTRE FOR MENTAL HEALTH, 2002

The forums included service users, carers, community organisations and statutory mental health representatives. The project team collected nominations from individuals and used these data to identify target audiences to work with over a 12-month period. The local police force was one target audience we identified and we approached them to see if they would be interested in receiving mental health awareness training.

> "*I became involved in the anti-stigma project because it is important that society begins to see mental health for what it really is, a health issue that needs addressing and not ignoring. Talking to the police is important because they are usually the ones who come into contact first hand with people in distress and how they deal with them initially can make all the difference.*" (Lisa Smith, member of Kent Awareness in Action).

The development of mental health awareness workshops has to be a consultative exercise because sessions must meet the training needs of the target group as well as the facilitators' agenda of addressing the stigma of mental illness. **Box 1** illustrates the process followed for developing workshops for Kent police.

BOX 1 Developing mental health awareness workshops

- Identify messages to communicate to the police through a series of focus group discussions with service users, carers and mental health professionals to explore their experiences of dealings with the police.
- Identify existing police mental health training resources (for example, National Schizophrenia Fellowship) and individuals with experience of mental health promotion to provide support and advice.
- Approach police forces with offer of mental health awareness workshops.
- Liaise with community liaison police officers to understand local policies, level of existing training provisions on mental health, identification of target audience (officers on patrol) and organise workshop session dates.
- Develop a baseline questionnaire to survey the mental health training needs of officers in two forces in Kent who were to receive our workshop programme (250 officers).
- Analyse data from police questionnaires to support the development of a workshop programme.
- Consult facilitators (both people working in the field of mental health and service users) involved in delivering the workshops to develop the workshop programme.
- Gain advice from community liaison police officers over the content of sessions before finalising the programme.

 © THE SAINSBURY CENTRE FOR MENTAL HEALTH, 2002

BOX 2 Miki's experience

Involving people in the community

"Like many people with mental health problems I have suffered as a result of people's pre-conceived ideas regarding mental illness, particularly the assumptions that my illness must mean that I am somehow not a worthwhile member of society and that I am incapable of intelligent thoughts or actions. I believe that many people think this way because they are ignorant of the real facts regarding mental illness and how it affects so many people's lives.

"Being involved in the project has allowed me to turn some very frustrating emotions into positive experiences. Hearing personal perspectives from service users will hopefully challenge the way some officers see mental illness and lead them to gain more of an understanding into how important their approach to someone suffering from mental distress is.

"However, having to stand up and speak about some very private emotions and situations is a bit like taking your clothes off in public. It is not easy and each time you do it, you are just as nervous as the last ... In my own mind I have balanced this out with the fact that I am doing this for a good reason, and I have nothing to feel ashamed of – an emotion that comes from the guilt of not being 'normal'."

(Miki Brunt, member of Kent Awareness in Action).

The police have been identified as an important and valuable service for people with mental health problems, particularly because they are accessible 24 hours a day. However, officers receive minimal mental health training.

The Police Complaints Authority has identified that training is needed to assist the police in their role of supporting people in mental distress including the use of section 136 of the *Mental Health Act 1983*, attending a victim of crime, and responding to a person making a suicide attempt. Communication between agencies involved in the care of people with mental health problems is a core standard of mental health modernisation programmes (Department of Health, 1998b), and the police are often involved with people with mental health problems, particularly outside normal office hours.

 © THE SAINSBURY CENTRE FOR MENTAL HEALTH, 2002

In the workshops, service users, people working in the field of mental health and police officers shared experiences, frustrations and points of good practice. An aim of the workshops was to value the role of the police and to demonstrate how important their approach actually is to an individual in distress.

Involvement of service users talking about personal issues was not always easy, as discussed above – there are personal risks associated with disclosure and projects have to consider the practical, emotional and structural barriers to participation in such initiatives, providing adequate training and support where necessary. It is also important that service users are not simply providing a token personal perspective in the sessions, but they are equal participants in the presentation team: One step away from the psychiatric system towards the mainstream:

> *"I hope that by reducing the stigma involved with mental health more opportunities will develop as people realise the input that people with mental health problems make is a valuable and unique contribution to society. My involvement in the police workshops will be a small step in a long journey."*
> (Piers Taylor, member of Kent Awareness in Action)

Educating people in the community

Information alone is insufficient support for the police in terms of providing officers with mental health awareness training. Lecturing that people with mental health problems are no more violent than the general public (Taylor and Gunn, 1999) will not be heard whilst police officers expectations and possibly experience work against the statistics.

In general, the police have a high level of understanding of mental health problems because officers deal with distressed people regularly in the course of their work, but what they did identify as training needs were specific skills to improve the services they provide to people with mental health problems (see **box 3**).

 © THE SAINSBURY CENTRE FOR MENTAL HEALTH, 2002

BOX 3 Police officers' ratings for the content of their workshops

What would you like the sessions to cover?	Respondents (212 officers)	
Local service provision and other support services	180	(85%)
Mental health law	156	(74%)
Sources of support for the police	153	(72%)
How to recognise mental distress	148	(70%)
Helping people who are suicidal	141	(67%)
Some understanding of how people with mental health problems feel	138	(65%)
Drugs, alcohol and mental health problems	125	(59%)
Helping people who are distressed	111	(52%)
Helping people who are angry	108	(51%)
Sources of additional information about mental health problems	86	(40%)

The workshop programme that we developed for Kent police borrowed material from the National Schizophrenia Fellowship police-training package and drew on the expertise of members of well-established local mental health awareness groups in Kent.

The project team developed a programme to ensure that each police officer in a training group received two workshops each lasting ninety minutes. An important part of the Awareness in Action programme is a comprehensive evaluation process, which we have yet to finish. This involves the completion of baseline and follow-up questionnaires, in addition to subjective evaluation ratings after each presentation.

The programme structure provided in **box 4** is therefore an outline guide to the approach we have adopted. We cannot describe effectiveness rating from the workshops at this stage in terms of the impact on police officers knowledge, understanding, attitudes or stated behaviour. Feedback from evaluation forms completed within the workshop sessions does reveal a very positive response to the programme with all officers stating that they have learnt something.

 © THE SAINSBURY CENTRE FOR MENTAL HEALTH, 2002

BOX 4 Mental health awareness workshops structure

- Aim to be interactive including a warm-up exercise, question and answer sessions, and discussion groups.
- Aim to be informative, enjoyable and challenging.
- Address officers' fears including addressing the link between violence, dangerousness and mental illness.
- Discuss frustrations with the mental health system and procedural difficulties at a local level.
- Hear personal perspectives of what it feels like when one is psychotic, depressed or distressed. Listen to personal accounts from a carer of how police involvement has helped a relative. Observe personal accounts of why a service user became involved with the police and what was helpful/unhelpful during their contact with them.
- Communication difficulties – attempt to simulate 'hearing voices' to crudely demonstrate the difficulties of communicating, thus promoting increased understanding and empathy.
- Dealing with distress – using case studies to explore how officers deal with an incident involving someone with a mental health problem, what other pressures are on them and how they might feel during and after the incident.
- Providing standards for good practice, which reinforce existing police practices for dealing with people in distress.
- Addressing the importance of nurturing one's own mental health highlighting that one in four people will experience mental health problems during the course of their lives.

 © THE SAINSBURY CENTRE FOR MENTAL HEALTH, 2002

A learning objective in the workshops is for the police to gain a better understanding of mental illness – the facts versus the myths – and to encourage officers to adopt more sensitive approaches for supporting people in distress. There are many procedural, structural and resource pressures on the police force and it is also important that our programme learns from officers' experiences, and adapts the workshops accordingly for future use.

Mental health awareness is here to stay

> *"This project is important to me, to go to people that play a vital part in the lives of service users, just for them to smile and not shuffle papers. It costs nothing to understand. Discrimination is a feeling of exclusion. It affects our health and happiness. It is very personal and in many cases it is unintended."*
> (Pat Still, member of Kent Awareness in Action)

Policy shifts and practical initiatives that focus on social capital (see article by Sarah Hean in ***Section Five*** of this resource), citizenship and social inclusion adopt a holistic approach for creating a healthy society. We all have responsibilities in creating and sustaining accepting communities but there is also a need for opportunities and choices in society to enable people to access valued roles.

Statutory and voluntary bodies have a stake in promoting the social inclusion of people with mental health problems. Stigma and discrimination do not have to be an inevitable consequence that accompanies a psychiatric diagnosis, but we are under no illusions over the difficulties faced even with the multitude of stigma intervention strategies that are emerging around the world.

Mental health awareness initiatives that promote changes in attitudes, understanding and behaviour towards people with mental health problems cannot exist in isolation from programmes that challenge societal value systems, political beliefs, education and economic systems, popular culture and the media. The foundation of mental health awareness programmes has to be longer lasting initiatives that can reinforce health promotion messages, alongside the initiatives that target specific community audiences.

 © THE SAINSBURY CENTRE FOR MENTAL HEALTH, 2002

Key points

- Which community audiences have been identified and offered mental health awareness training in the past year? How have service users been involved in selecting suitable audiences?
- Ask service users about their experiences of the target audience and identify the main messages. Do you have practical suggestions to make about how people can support the inclusion of people with mental health difficulties? Have other groups already created suitable resources that you could use? How will service users contribute to the design and delivery of the training?
- Identify one or more allies in the target audience who will help to formulate the training and support the practical arrangements.
- Find out what the community audience already knows. Have they received training? Do their policies support full citizenship for people with mental health problems? Have there been specific problems in the past? How do they view training? What would they like a session to cover?
- How will you evaluate the success of the training event?

© THE SAINSBURY CENTRE FOR MENTAL HEALTH, 2002

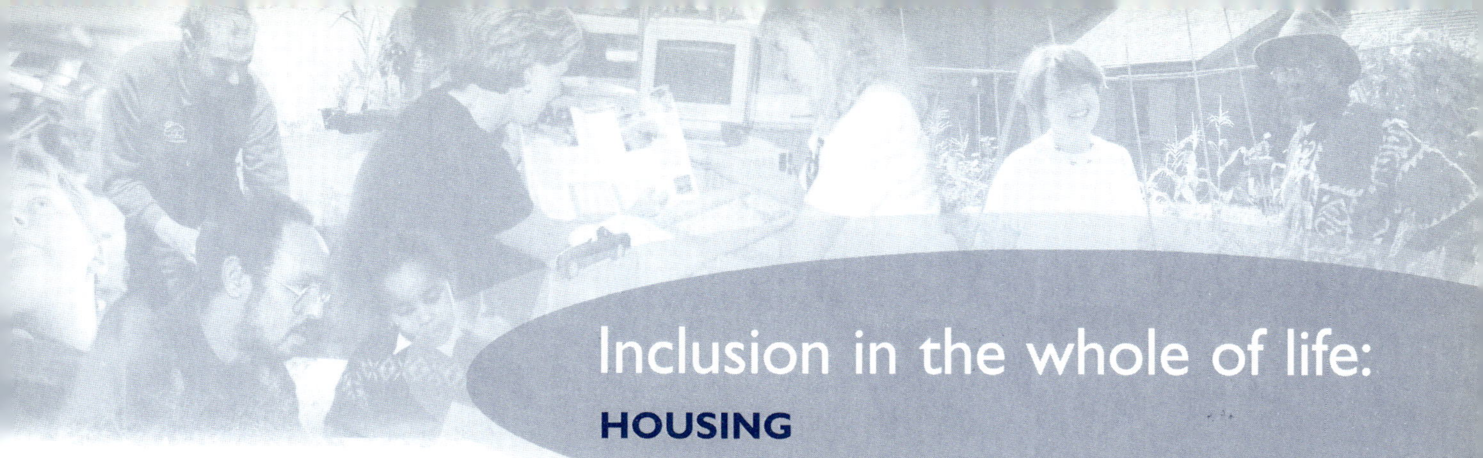

Inclusion in the whole of life:
HOUSING

LIBRARY
CHARLES FREARS CAMPUS
DE MONTFORT UNIVERSITY

Maurice Harker

The closure of long stay institutions and the development of community care have brought housing forward as a key element of the new solutions and possibilities available for people with mental health problems. Some needs identified from a local study (Jones and Kent, 1997) are listed here:

- Significant numbers of people with mental health problems living in hostels for homeless people where staffing and support regimes are unlikely to be adequate.
- A person previously living independently often found him or herself unable to cope which may have resulted in moves to acute hospitals, hostels or the street.
- There is evidence that discharge from hospitals, both acute and non acute, is delayed because the required level of support or funding for care in the community is not available and there is a shortage of independent accommodation of a sufficient standard with appropriate levels of floating support.
- There is a need for expansion of specialist provision to provide medium to high levels of assistance.

Early stages for housing services

Initially the alternatives to institutions took two forms – well-staffed therapeutic community projects and group homes where small numbers of single people shared in ordinary housing usually with more limited staff support. In the early 1980s, the Department of the Environment commissioned research on 'housing for mentally ill and mentally handicapped people' (Ritchie and Keegan, 1983). This study provides a benchmark against which we can chart changes in the scale, range and patterns of funding for supported housing provision available to people with learning disabilities and people with mental health problems.

Since 1983 there has been a marked increase in the overall number of community-based supported housing schemes. There were large variations then, as now, in the scale and range of housing and support services in different regions and a similar pattern of predominantly urban provision.

Unstaffed group homes formed the major part of the provision in the mid 1980s. Local authorities ran these group homes, usually offering a low to moderate level of support, with a heavy reliance on input of support services from the voluntary sector. Housing associations at that time provided just over 30% of the accommodation and most of the rest were council tenancies.

Following the introduction of the *NHS and Community Care Act 1990* and the loosening, in the early 1990s, of Housing Corporation restrictions on what constituted 'special needs' provision, services have become much more diverse. Individual care packages and floating support services have become significant features, as has the wider use of mainstream housing within the social rented sector. There is also increased awareness of the need to provide support services that can range across tenures. As predicted by the 1983 report, housing and support providers have redirected their services to offer more self-contained accommodation, including clustered, self-contained flats.

Persistent problems

The 1983 report expressed concerns in a number of areas, some of which still remain to be properly addressed today. They included the following:

- a lack of a coherent framework for housing and support options, with evidence of short-term approaches to dealing with problems of funding and resource management;
- the lack of involvement at a strategic level of local authority housing departments in relation to community-based provision;
- evidence of mismatch between the types of services available and the expressed needs of people with mental health problems;
- an increase in scale and activity does not, of itself, guarantee improvements in quality and effectiveness;
- the lack of central and local information on supported housing schemes, which makes it difficult to review and plan for the future.

Government policy

In 1998, *Modernising Social Services* (Department of Health, 1998a) stated that the aims and objectives for services should be:

- To promote the independence of adults assessed as needing social care support arranged by the local authority, respecting their dignity and furthering their social and economic participation.

 © THE SAINSBURY CENTRE FOR MENTAL HEALTH, 2002

- To enable adults assessed as needing social care support to live as safe, full and as normal a life as possible, in their own home wherever feasible.
- To plan, commission, purchase and monitor an adequate supply of appropriate, cost effective and safe social care provision for those eligible for local authority support.
- To identify individuals with social care needs who are eligible for public support, to assess those needs accurately and consistently, and to review care packages as necessary to ensure that they continue to be appropriate and effective.

This was followed by more detailed recommendations in the 1998 White Paper on mental health services (Department of Health, 1998b). This set out a programme of reform for mental health care in England and Wales and outlines the principles and strategy required to improve the way that services respond to people with mental illness. The document states:

> *"Dealing with social exclusion is central to tackling the root causes of illness... Difficulties in finding and sustaining work, and in obtaining adequate financial support are characteristic of those who are socially excluded and a particular problem for those with mental illness.*
>
> *"A modern mental health service will provide care which is integrated and which is focused on the individual, recognising that different people have different needs and preferences. It will be evidence-based and outcome-driven. Services will be there for people when they need them and where they need them. Services must be safe, sound and supportive."*

The *National Service Framework For Mental Health* (Department of Health, 1999b) translates these principles into seven standards and then sets out how these standards will be implemented. Implications for the provision of local housing and support services include the following key points:

- better use of 'assertive outreach' services;
- improved population needs assessment for service planning and as part of health improvement programmes;
- sufficient community-based 24-hour staffed facilities;
- good risk management and investment in crisis responses;
- a mental health grant is also made available, dependent on approval of local authority expenditure plans.

Proposals were made for the co-ordination of services to achieve improved risk management through joint working and the integration of health and social services assessment approaches into one system, the care programme approach (Department of Health, 1999a).

Guidance was given in 1992 and 1997 jointly by the Department of Health and the Department of the Environment in local authority circulars and a workbook on housing

 © THE SAINSBURY CENTRE FOR MENTAL HEALTH, 2002

and community care, encouraging joint planning and joint assessment (Department of the Environment and Department of Health, 1997).

More recently, the *Local Government Bill 1999* included a new power for local authorities to manage and distribute a specific grant for welfare and support services. This follows from the proposals in the consultation document *Supporting People* (1998) to create a local authority budget to replace funds for support currently provided through housing benefit, the Housing Corporation's Supported Housing Management Grant and grants from the probation service. A 'Supporting People Grant' specifically for the purpose of funding support will be administered by local authorities. Key features of the grant are:

- to promote independence, to prevent people from having to enter more institutional settings, and to assist with re-settlement in the community;
- it will not be tied to property but focused on people;
- it will be distributed to local authorities on the basis of an index of support needs;
- it will be a single, co-ordinated budget for support needs;
- there will be incentives to promote value for money and independent monitoring and inspection.

A 'Supporting People' plan will be produced locally which must:

- map needs and supply, including specific reference to minority ethnic needs;
- review performance;
- take account of users' views;
- link into other strategic plans such as health improvement plans, housing strategies, community care plans and crime and disorder strategies;
- set aims and priorities by client group;
- define 'cross-authority' arrangements;
- lay out adequate commissioning, monitoring and review arrangements at scheme level.

Organisation around individual needs

The government's modernising theme for the future of public services encompasses and promotes giving people a choice in the kinds of services available and how they get them. While there is sometimes resistance to detailed strategic planning on the grounds that service development should always centre on individual needs and preferences, in practice the two levels of planning are interdependent. Without the perspective of individual needs, strategic planning can easily become too managerial and service focused.

© THE SAINSBURY CENTRE FOR MENTAL HEALTH, 2002

With regard to housing and support, people should be able to get the support services they require without having to move into a particular form of accommodation. While this may not always be possible where support needs are very intensive or where there are needs for certain types of therapeutic support or rehabilitation, the principle holds for the great majority of people with mental health problems living in the community.

The other side of the coin is that people should have the opportunity to move into a particular scheme or type of accommodation if this is what they need and want. There are many areas of the country where supported housing is in very short supply and people with severe mental health problems have no choice but to try and survive in independent housing with minimal support. At its worst this problem manifests itself in large numbers of people with mental illness staying in homelessness hostels or on acute psychiatric wards because there is no suitable accommodation for them.

Hurdles faced by people seeking housing and support

It is usually difficult to get information about what is already available in the area and what other options may be feasible. There can be very limited choice in types of services or where they are located. Various bureaucratic obstacles and tests may need to be passed, including formal needs assessment or the allocation of points for housing.

Funding has to be negotiated with one or more agencies and its effects on personal disposable income understood. Practical arrangements may have to be made, such as furnishing and decorating a property. An individual care/support plan may need to be agreed with the support agency.

Classification of types of housing

What has been apparent in housing and support for people over the last 20 years is growing diversity. There is now more choice and a preference for less institutional settings. This can be described in terms of two dimensions – form of housing and nature of support (King and Harker, 2000).

Gradually more possibilities have been added to each dimension; we have been putting more points on the continuum of care and housing as illustrated in **box 1**. There is a tendency as you move from bottom left to top right to increase the individual's independence, choice and personal control. The types of accommodation or support identified on each axis are for illustration only – this is not a comprehensive list.

 © THE SAINSBURY CENTRE FOR MENTAL HEALTH, 2002

BOX 1 Housing and care continuum

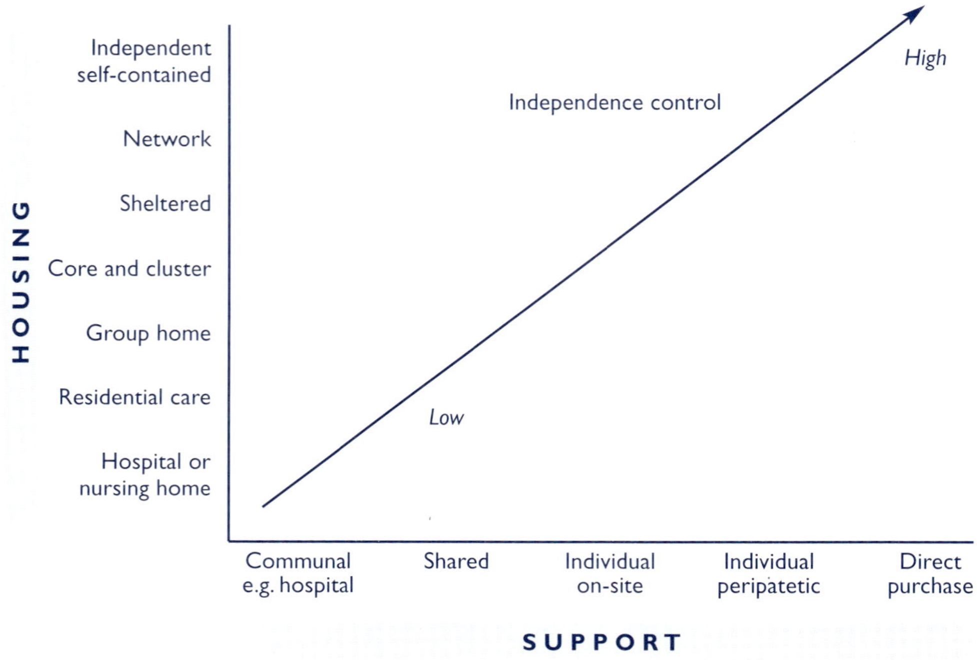

Source: *Making Housing Choices*

While the graph shows seven main types of housing and five types of support, these may be divided into further sub-categories.

Pick and mix

As explained, housing is only one dimension of a support service and it is increasingly possible to 'pick and mix' different combinations of the variables outlined in **box 1** – and other variables as well – so a service is designed for an individual. Lynn Watson uses five variables in recent Joseph Rowntree research (see **box 2**) generating (in theory) 7,776 options (Watson and Tarpey, 1998). Clearly not all of these options are practical.

BOX 2 Pick and mix

Housing and support services				
Pick and mix – select your types				
Housing type	***Support type***	***Support level***	***Management and finances***	***Tenure***
Self-contained independent	Individual service package	High/intensive long-term	User managed with direct payments	Mixed – owned and rented/ owned
Locality/area network	Visiting designated team/worker	Low/medium long-term	Grant funded or block purchasing	Rented – local authority
Single site cluster	Adjacent/on-site staff	High/intensive fluctuating	Service charge/tenant contributions	Rented – housing association
Small shared (2/3 people)	Integral staff night/sleep in	Medium/high increasing	Individual care packages	Mixed – rented private/social housing
Large shared (4+ people)	Integral staff Day/office base	High/intensive reducing	Voluntary/ private residential home fees	Licence – statutory/ voluntary/ private care agency
Placement/ lodgings	Live-in carer/support worker	Low/medium reducing	Statutory run and financed service	Rented – private landlord

'Pick and Mix' (Watson and Tarpey, 1998).

What is needed now?

Provision remains inadequate for:

- people with multiple needs, such as those with drug or alcohol problems and mentally ill offenders;
- people in crisis and those with episodic high care needs;
- intensive support, 24-hour supervision;
- active programmes of skills development and rehabilitation.

The gulf between hospital and community housing projects is still wide. People often get stuck in hospital, at home or in hostels. Social services cannot afford to provide the necessary volume of high quality care.

 © THE SAINSBURY CENTRE FOR MENTAL HEALTH, 2002

More accommodation in networks or clusters of self-contained supported housing is wanted. Housing providers want support for people to sustain their tenancy and avoid breakdown and help with resettlement into a home from hospital or hostel.

Some local authorities think there are too many large registered care homes and that some people with lower support needs could manage without full time staffing. Small group homes are no longer being commissioned to any great extent and there is a recurring difficulty with filling vacancies as they arise.

Although housing and support services may be provided separately they need to be planned together so that the supply of both are managed as part of a single package. If the support is weak the tenancy may fail, while if suitable housing is not available the stability will be missing from a support service. Housing, health care and social support must to be planned and managed together – the original premise for community care – and this remains all too rare.

Key points

- Map the accommodation options in your area. You may wish to generate a number of useful options from the 'pick and mix' table and then check how many places of each type are available in your local area. Does the supply match the need?
- Can people get the support they need without moving into a particular kind of accommodation?
- What action is being taken in relation to homeless people with mental health difficulties in your area?
- Do housing providers think that health care, social support and housing are well co-ordinated in your area?
- Who decides how your 'Supporting People' grant is spent?
- How are (a) service users, and (b) representatives of ethnic minority communities involved in developing the 'Supporting People' plan?

© THE SAINSBURY CENTRE FOR MENTAL HEALTH, 2002

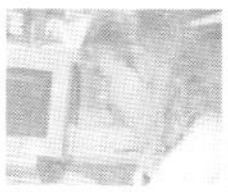

Case Study

Developing a supported living service for people with enduring mental illness

Southern Focus Trust has developed a network of community-based services for people with enduring mental illness in Fareham and Gosport. This has demonstrated how flexibility and open working with clients has been able to meet the changing needs of people with enduring mental illness. The flexibility of the service has meant that residents have been able to remain in their home as their needs change, and admission to hospital has been prevented.

Background to the service development

The first services that were provided as a final stepping-stone for those leaving hospital, and as a pathway towards independent living, were group homes. A resettlement service was also developed. This was to prevent homelessness and re-admissions to hospital through inadequate housing and support to those in the community.

One solution to this problem was a scheme whereby the council sublet properties to the Trust, which would then let the property to people identified by social and health services as needing support in establishing themselves in the community. Over time, with support, the aim was for these tenants to revert to an ordinary council tenancy. Other similar supported tenancies were also added to this service.

Supported living service

At first separate services were developed, each with its own staffing structure linking in with the larger psychiatric services. It began to be recognised that although this provided an adequate patchwork of services, in mental health services in particular people's needs change regularly. When unwell, a person may need a lot of support, but when well they may need only a little support. In all there was a realisation that the service needed to be knitted together into a more comprehensive and flexible system.

The 'supported living' model was adopted with the following aims and values:

- A person-centred approach should be adopted, providing what people both needed and wanted, rather than fitting the person into the existing structure of the service.
- The service needed to be flexible, so that it could change with the changing needs of the recipients.
- Support should be innovative and creative and enable people to develop relationships of their choice both in and out of the service.

 © THE SAINSBURY CENTRE FOR MENTAL HEALTH, 2002

- The service should offer a continuum of support so that people can move to more independence should their needs change. A system where the level of support depends upon the changing needs of the residents has meant there has had to be more involvement in the co-ordination and management of support.
- Care must also be taken to link staff with specific clients when this is needed as the service users have placed importance on being supported by staff they know and trust, particularly when they are going through difficult periods.
- Regular reviews of individual needs are essential and greater management co-ordination and evaluation is required than was necessary under the fixed staffing system.
- Greater inter-agency liaison is needed to ensure that the service provided as a whole is working to agreed objectives.
- The care programme approach is vital to involve everyone with the client in identifying the service and support needs to be met.

BOX 3 The supported living model

Management structure

The management structure was changed so that the whole service came under one manager and the staffing structure was changed to provide more flexibility within the service. A team of staff providing support across the shared houses and various tenancies was brought together so that when needs changed the support could be targeted to where it was needed. Having a floating team means that if a resident moves to another part of the service there can be some continuity in staff contact.

How we did it

Through the care programme approach we were able to work with the residents to identify areas of their lives where they would need support, the number of hours involved and when help would be given. After a few weeks in operation this was again reviewed, as one of the residents was feeling very insecure having been in a high care environment for so many years.

We were able to increase the support particularly at those times when residents were most vulnerable and indeed on one occasion when there was a crisis he was able to have one of the staff sleep over at the house. We were therefore able to overcome this difficult period and now four months later have been able to reduce the number of support hours with the agreement of the resident.

© THE SAINSBURY CENTRE FOR MENTAL HEALTH, 2002

Key points

Our experience in setting up this supported living service has demonstrated how flexibility and open working with our clients has been able to meet the changing needs of people with enduring mental illness. Success depends on a trusting relationship between the staff and service users and close working relationships with the statutory services.

More focused management is also required with a greater proportion of time being spent on planning the allocation of staff hours and service user contact time. The flexibility of the service has meant that residents have been able to remain in their homes as their needs change and hospital admission is prevented.

Overall, the service has gone a long way in meeting the objectives and there have been some lessons learned along the way.

 © THE SAINSBURY CENTRE FOR MENTAL HEALTH, 2002

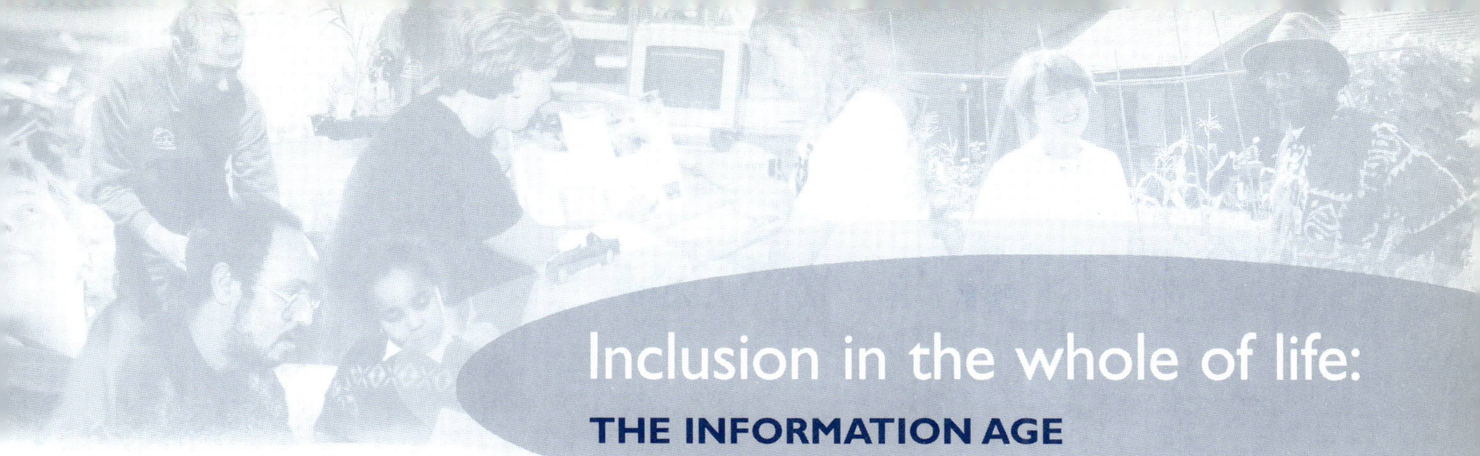

Inclusion in the whole of life:
THE INFORMATION AGE

Melba Wilson

In 1998, Mind undertook an inquiry whose focus was to ascertain the degree of exclusion experienced by people with mental health problems. The 12-month Creating Accepting Communities Inquiry aimed to gather and consider evidence on mental health and social exclusion from a wide range of individuals, groups and organisations. These ranged from high-street retailers to individual service users, and NHS trusts to small voluntary groups, including black and minority ethnic groups.

The Inquiry found:

> "*...mounting evidence of the discrimination experienced by people with mental health problems in Britain. This discrimination results in their systematic exclusion from society. Social exclusion operates in all areas of life – daily living, work and training, and access to services, including health, financial, consumer and leisure services.*" (Dunn, 1999).

It also found that exclusion was a compound process – exclusion in one area of life often leads to exclusion in other areas. One witness commented:

> "*Psychiatry has created such fear of people who have mental health problems. Those who have had mental health problems have been traditionally regarded as the lowest of the low. Unemployment, social isolation, poverty, homelessness, stigma, contempt and fear surround people with mental health problems like a shroud. It is easier to live in society with a prison record than a psychiatric record.*" (Hywel Davies, Pembrokeshire Hearing Voices Group. Witness to Creating Accepting Communities Inquiry).

Examples of the exclusion of mental health service users came up in every sphere of public and private life – from difficulties in getting a driving licence or booking a holiday to discriminatory attitudes from insurers, through to barriers blocking access to health care or employment.

 © THE SAINSBURY CENTRE FOR MENTAL HEALTH, 2002

From exclusion to inclusion

> "*Social inclusion must come down surely to somewhere to live, something to do, someone to love. It's as simple – and as complicated – as that. There are all kinds of barriers to people with mental health problems having those three things.*" (Charles Fraser, St. Mungo's, Witness to Mind's Inquiry on Creating Accepting Communities).

Ten guiding principles for social inclusion

The Mind Inquiry identified ten principles of social inclusion. They are:

1. A healthy society maximises opportunity for each of its members, regardless of their circumstances.
2. A healthy society is also one that embraces diversity and is not threatened by cultures, beliefs or behaviours outside society's norms.
3. Nobody is a 'burden' on society. Everyone is part of society and has an inherent and absolute worth as a human being.
4. Promoting social inclusion involves the active fostering of the mutual inter-dependence between individuals, groups of people and the state.
5. The social exclusion of any group of people creates schisms that are bad not only for the mental health of excluded individuals but also for the mental health of society as a whole.
6. Social exclusion is a 'compound' process. Its inter-connections mean exclusion in one area of life often leads to exclusion in another.
7. Inclusion therefore needs to be addressed in a holistic way. The catalysts that promote inclusion will have wide-ranging benefits for individuals and communities.
8. Specialist services must be conceived as stepping-stones to inclusion, not departure points for exclusion. The ultimate aim of inclusion is enabling participation in the mainstream of society for all those who desire it.
9. Excluded groups are experts by experience. All processes of consultation, policy-making and practice must not just include, but be driven by the views and needs of excluded groups.
10. Promoting inclusion means leading public opinion. Clear and consistent messages from government, public bodies and the voluntary sector are the only way to tackle 'them and us' thinking.

 © THE SAINSBURY CENTRE FOR MENTAL HEALTH, 2002

Aims of social inclusion

Mind's work on social inclusion takes these guiding principles as its starting point. The aim is to shift the focus from the exclusion of people with mental health problems, through developing practical solutions and outcomes to promote their social inclusion.

It is being undertaken in the context of working within a broad spectrum that includes, but is not limited to, initiatives which are specifically related to mental health. The approach is to build upon the outcomes and recommendations of the Inquiry report to create holistic and integrated frameworks for inclusion.

The goal is to develop and pilot workable and measurable models of service provision and infrastructure across a range of sectors, the purpose of which is to improve the quality of life for people with long-term mental health problems. Projects need to be sustainable and transferable. The work involves seeking and sustaining practical partnerships across sectors – including health, mental health, local authority, education, community groups and users of mental health services.

The intention is to create flexible models to be used by local authorities, education and employment bodies, as well as public health and mental health services. The models will incorporate clinical and non-clinical outcomes; develop measures in the areas of discrimination prevention, effective partnerships, physical and mental health improvement, and enabling fair access to opportunities. Specific foci are on race and culture; the arts and sport; employment; education and training; and neighbourhood inclusion.

Local circumstances dictate both the direction and the content of the pilot projects. Currently, Mind has set up one pilot site in the London Borough of Merton. The focus here is on employment. It is also setting up a series of long-term pilots in Wales. The first of these will have a focus on arts, education and leisure, and is being developed in partnership with Caerphilly County Borough Council, South Wales.

 © THE SAINSBURY CENTRE FOR MENTAL HEALTH, 2002

Case Study London Borough of Merton Pilot (Cyber Café Project)

Aim

The project aims to promote employment prospects, leisure interests and greater access to higher education for mental health service users in the London Borough of Merton. The focus is on enabling internet access, through information and training.

The project will:

- enable internet access;
- enable mental health service users to develop IT skills;
- promote leisure;
- promote employment by developing a website where mental health service users can share information about the skills they offer, and prospective employers can advertise local job vacancies;
- develop local information provision;
- provide IT training for staff and users.

Duration of pilot

The Merton project is a 12-month pilot, which began in January 2001. It is important to note, however, that a key expected outcome is the identification of long-term resources and relationships for sustaining and further developing the initiative.

Scope of pilot

The Merton pilot encompasses work with seven day centres in Merton. A range of statutory and voluntary sector service providers including Merton Social Services, Merton Mind, and Richmond Fellowship run the day centres. The diverse client base includes black and minority ethnic service users, elderly service users, as well as service users generally covered within the context of the *National Service Framework for Mental Health* (Department of Health, 1999b) – i.e. working age adults to age 65.

Partnership

As noted earlier, the Creating Accepting Communities pilots are being undertaken in the context of developing and sustaining local partnerships. The partners in the Merton pilot project are: Mind, Disability Alliance Merton (comprising Merton Mind and its day centres),

Merton Social Services, Merton College and Pathfinder User Employment Project. This represents a broad mix of statutory and voluntary sector provision, and is a good basis for engaging with a broad spectrum of mental health service users.

Monitoring

A steering / working group, which includes users of mental health services and partner representatives, guides the Cyber Café Project. The group works with the project co-ordinator to troubleshoot, keep track of the day-to-day work, and identify opportunities and outcomes for further development and integration.

User feedback

Obtaining the feedback of service users is an important aspect of the work. User expectations and the extent to which the project meets them will be constantly assessed throughout the life of the project. This will take the form of questionnaires, and periodic assessment, involving one-to-one and group feedback between service users, the project co-ordinator and the partners.

Partner contributions

The successful development and progression of the Cyber Café Project is in part due to identifying: (a) the contributions that each partner can make and (b) the outcomes which each expects. The project has learned that it is important to ensure there is clarity about each at the outset. **Box 1** sets out the contributions and outcomes for the main partners in Merton.

 © THE SAINSBURY CENTRE FOR MENTAL HEALTH, 2002

BOX 1 Merton Cyber Café Project

Partnership contributions	Desirable outcomes
Disability Alliance Merton • sites • access to mental health service users; • financial and human resources.	**Disability Alliance Merton** • greater access and skills development for client groups; • greater information sharing about provision of local services; • agencies and initiatives.
Mind • develop pilot in context of partnership working; • disseminate outcomes; • contribute resources to the initiative budget; • recruit and supervise a project co-ordinator; • monitor the progress of the work with regard to timetable and focus; • act as the secretariat for the project.	**Mind** • development of Phase II work on social inclusion to include demonstrable gains and outcomes through the development of workable and transferable models of social inclusion.
Merton College • launch site for the project; • training expertise; • IT and technical support – including trouble shooting and telephone support.	**Merton College** • promotion of greater access to mainstream courses for people with mental health problems.
Pathfinder User Employment Project • access to information on prospective employment within the local mental health trust (South West London & St. George's Mental Health NHS Trust).	**Pathfinder User Employment Project** • increased access to employment for service users in the Trust's client population.

© THE SAINSBURY CENTRE FOR MENTAL HEALTH, 2002

Partnership

The work began by building consensus on the way forward, identifying goals and creating a written agreement between partners. Recognition of the fact that clients can also be partners was also a crucial step to building ownership of the project.

The keys to strong partnership are:

- a diverse range of partners, including health authorities, higher education, local charities, user groups and local government;
- equal treatment of all involved, be they clients, funders or advisers;
- regular consultation, discussion and information sharing;
- transparent objectives with clear indicators of progress.

Barriers to partnership

The range of partners can mean that keeping all partners informed, aware and in contact can be difficult within limited resources, especially time. Email is a quick and cost effective way to address this problem, if all partners have this facility!

Participation

Monthly reports, quarterly meetings and day-to-day contact mean that partners are aware, informed and regularly inputting into the process of building the project. 'Piggy-backing' on existing networks can be a key step to building trust and credibility for the project, especially with clients.

The keys to ensuring wide and worthwhile participation are:

- to tap into existing networks;
- ensure openness and easy channels for communication;
- encourage mutual trust and reliance.

Obstacles to participation

Key obstacles to participation include: lack of information; use of difficult, non-accessible language; lack of compensation to service users for their time; a failure to challenge stigmatising terms; inadequate administration, including lack of timely provision of information and under-representation of some the parties. Any of these obstacles will consistently block ownership and therefore participation. Avoiding such errors is helped by making awareness raising a key part of the work, and by having the resources to address the issues.

The experience of the Merton pilot is that there is a high degree of understanding, commitment and involvement. This helps to: create a willingness to seek a shared understanding; promote the active engagement of mental health service users, and engender a focus on sustaining the work in the long term.

Expected outcomes

Practical

- production of a manual on basic computer skills and a guide to the internet;
- project transfer guidelines;
- development of a socially inclusive website for mental health service users;
- guidelines for use of the internet by vulnerable people.

Intangibles

- goodwill, development of local and national contacts and partnerships, i.e. between national Mind and the local Mind association, mental health service users, local college, local government and health trust;
- sharing of good practice between partners and more widely (i.e. nationally). A forum for service users to share their knowledge and experience of the mental health system;
- perceptible improvement in quality of life for service users.

Conclusion

Mind is concerned that issues of stigma, poverty and discrimination, which result in the social exclusion of people with mental health problems, should be replaced with a shared understanding and emphasis on mental health promotion, access to care, services and opportunities to promote social inclusion. The need to engage local people in finding local solutions – not least mental health service users – is integral.

Mind's social inclusion initiative – through the Creating Accepting Communities pilots – is demonstrably well placed to help generate good outcomes that will make a difference to the lives of people with long-term mental health problems. The work is underpinned by principles of choice, participation, dignity and respect. Mind believes that this makes for a good combination for inclusion.

 © THE SAINSBURY CENTRE FOR MENTAL HEALTH, 2002

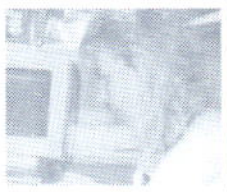

Case Study Jacques' story

In Merton, seven organisations are participating in a project to promote employment prospects, leisure opportunities and provide training places to mental health service users, by giving them internet access and then promoting these opportunities through the project website.

The following case study represents a composite example of how this project has been working, and gives insight into the issues that can arise. We have changed some names, details and events to protect the privacy of those involved.

Jacques has a mental health problem. He has spent three years in hospital and on leaving was referred to the local day centre which he has been attending for the last two years. He finds the facilities useful and has many long-standing friends, whom he goes there to meet. He is already participating in some voluntary work to help out at a local charity and finds the work rewarding.

In our experience of setting up and promoting the Cyber Café Project, we found that initially people are worried that they are being pushed into doing something they do not want to do. They may be worried about making themselves look silly, or at not being able to do something, supposedly easy enough for a child to pick up.

Despite this, Jacques decides, after watching some friends, and with a bit of encouragement, to give it a go. He reasons that the local user project has much of its most up-to-date information on the computer 'somewhere' and it seems to be the 'way forward.' He has also found himself increasing unable to relate to his 12-year-old grandson who is always 'going on about the internet.'

Initially many of the tools – ways of navigating and the internet environment – seem difficult to use and almost like a different culture or world. He perseveres and eventually starts to find some useful tools, e.g. email and catching up with the news. The project co-ordinator proposes a formal course, which will give people who have been using the project a recognised qualification.

Jacques notices that many people are already signed up and decides to give it a go, once a week at the local college. Through the college he meets many people who are in the same position, who have been working their way though many of the same problems he has. He finds it a useful forum which provides a way for him to bounce his ideas off other people.

Jacques is now considering what further courses he may want to take up at the college and has been thinking about what he can do with his skills at a local level.

 © THE SAINSBURY CENTRE FOR MENTAL HEALTH, 2002

Key points

At Mind

- People with experience of mental distress were surveyed to find out how social exclusion has affected their lives.
- New projects must be sustainable and transferable.
- One of the project aims is to support people to engage in leisure activities in the wider community.
- The contribution and expected outcome for each partner was set out clearly.
- The need to communicate with partners was recognised as important and existing networks were used wherever possible.

© THE SAINSBURY CENTRE FOR MENTAL HEALTH, 2002

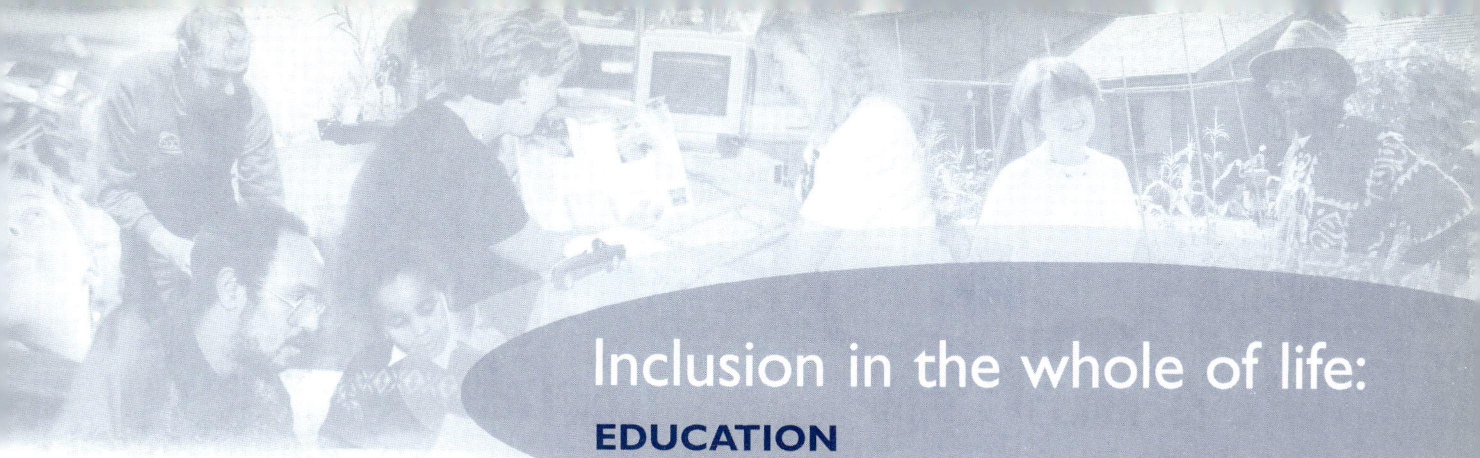

Inclusion in the whole of life:
EDUCATION

Kathryn James and Jacqueline Henderson

> *"In the past I suffered from depression and stress, mainly because of lack of self-accomplishment and poor education. Filling these empty areas of my life with learning has opened up a new life for me. I am a more relaxed, happier person and more at ease with people and equal to others, fully able to stand up for myself and speak for myself."* (Student).

In the past few years many providers of adult, further and community education have actively sought to encourage participation in learning for people who experience mental health difficulties. The publication of the Tomlinson (1996) report urged learning providers to move beyond the labels that are attached to people on to a more inclusive approach. Providers were encouraged to enable people to learn by creating appropriate learning environments and looking for the best fit between an individual's learning requirements and the provision that is made for them.

Importantly, it also noted that traditionally mental health service users had been excluded from education. In 1997 the Further Education Funding Council report (Kennedy 1997) promoted education as a weapon against poverty, isolation and exclusion and saw it as a route to participation and active citizenship. The report states that: *"Equity dictates that all should have the right to succeed."*

The *National Service Framework for Mental Health* (Department of Health, 1999b) has at its heart seven standards, of which mental health promotion is number one. The standard makes the link between adverse life conditions and poor mental health. While no specific mention is made about links to adult education, education can be a route out of poverty as well as having many social benefits and opportunities for personal development and growth.

This article is intended for managers and practitioners in mental health services who want to develop local learning opportunities for people with mental health difficulties. We suggest ways in which you can support your local learning provider and identify factors they should be considering when they establish or evaluate educational provision.

 © THE SAINSBURY CENTRE FOR MENTAL HEALTH, 2002

Partnership

Undoubtedly the most successful provision for mental health service users is based on a foundation of strong partnership between the learning providers and mental health services. Even better is a three-way partnership that includes service users who have a say in the development of educational opportunities. Ways of establishing collaborative working could include:

- Setting up a steering group or advisory group where issues can be discussed and problems solved. The advisory group at one college discussed issues such as the appropriate level of support for learners. They went on to produce an information sheet for students and referrers on what students could expect from college and what might be expected from them. This helped students, tutors and mental health service practitioners to decide what kind of learning opportunity was appropriate for an individual. Students with mental health difficulties were included in this group and their expenses paid so they could attend.
- Some students may not feel comfortable in attending a formal meeting like an advisory group. It can help to support students to meet together in the absence of college staff to discuss issues that are then reported back to the college. Students may gain a great sense of empowerment by having a mechanism through which their voice is heard and also by establishing a system of peer support within the learning environment.
- It is worth devoting some time to discussing the aim of each learning opportunity. For example, one course may aim to enhance the quality of people's daily experience at a day centre while another may give people confidence and skills to move on and use other community facilities. Arriving at a shared understanding of the purpose of a learning opportunity will help to specify the arrangements.
- Many learning providers consider this to be new ground and making judgements on what information is required about a student, what level of support is necessary or what to do in a crisis can be more fraught than it needs to be. Some practitioners in education will need reassurance that they do not need specialist knowledge about mental health or be privy to certain information about individuals, and that crises rarely happen. Most education staff will value the support of mental health practitioners as they set up procedures and establish good practice with regard to confidentiality, boundaries and in encouraging independence in learners.
- Some mental health service providers have provided supervision or mentorship to those education staff that work closely with students who have mental health difficulties. Again, this can be essential in ensuring good practice and supporting the staff member in a demanding area of work.

 © THE SAINSBURY CENTRE FOR MENTAL HEALTH, 2002

Staff development

Staff working in further, adult and community education reflect the same range of views and opinions about mental health as the general public. Work may have to be done to enable a learning provider to create a more accepting environment.

- Mental health practitioners can assist by providing mental health awareness sessions to all education staff – canteen staff and caretakers as well as tutors, support staff and managers. Presentations from students can be particularly powerful.
- Events such as World Mental Health Day provide an opportunity jointly to plan activities for all students and staff in further and adult education. Such events celebrate the work and achievement of mental health service users and can also help to remove the stigma around mental ill health.
- Staff in mental health services may also need their awareness raising. They may not be aware of the great changes that have taken place in adult, community and further education in the past few years, the opportunities that are available or the impact that learning can have on a person. Some colleges have open days or visits for mental health service staff in order to show them the variety and flexibility of the learning opportunities on offer. This also helps mental health staff to talk to service users about the possibility of returning to education.

Accessing learning opportunities

> *"I have gained confidence and I feel more in control, which in turn reduces the level of stress and depression. I can see a way forward, getting off the treadmill and back to contributing to society. Even if it is a long way ahead of me at least I know that the chance is there to be taken. I feel more on a level with my peers, most of whom have had families and most have returned back to work."* (Student)

In setting up provision, learning providers need to give careful consideration to how they enable students to access learning opportunities. It is almost too obvious to point out that there is no typical student with mental health difficulties; each individual will have a different experience of mental health that may or may not affect their learning. They will also have different experiences of education, different abilities and different interests. So while courses set up specifically for mental health service users can meet some needs, learning providers also need to think about how they can meet individual needs.

 © THE SAINSBURY CENTRE FOR MENTAL HEALTH, 2002

A named contact

Most learning providers that have successfully encouraged participation of mental health service users in their organisations have a designated person to whom mental health practitioners can refer and who, when students have started at college, is their named person to contact for ongoing support and guidance.

The role of the named person can be to:

- make initial contact with mental health services by talking to staff about what is on offer and how to refer people;
- provide one-to-one guidance to service users about what learning they may want and how they can best be supported to access it;
- provide one-to-one support to individuals after enrolment at college to discuss progression on to other learning programmes or how to manage a break from learning arising from illness or other commitments.

Some colleges have identified existing members of staff for this role or recruited a person specifically for it. Alternatively, other colleges have seconded a person from health services (perhaps an occupational therapist) to fulfil this valuable role (see **box 1**). There are advantages and disadvantages to each of these options.

The named person will have a guidance role to work with individuals. Where there have been good examples of this role working effectively the guidance has been:

- centred on what the individual wants to learn and enjoys doing rather than starting from a 'deficit model' of what they need to improve;
- delivered in the place where the individual feels most comfortable, for example, in a day centre, community mental health team venue, at college or even in their own home;
- is not time-limited, as some individuals may need more than one meeting to discuss their aims and needs;
- is practical and may involve visits to different learning venues, meeting a tutor or even sitting in a canteen before a student can make an informed decision about which learning opportunity is best for them;
- tailored to include and support individuals who prefer mainstream learning programmes rather than specialist courses for mental health service users. Time can be spent with them to identify the right course and the level of support they may need.

Time spent at this stage often means that the person will choose the right course for them, one in which they can be as independent as possible and will know what to expect. This mitigates as far as possible against the hazard of being on the wrong course that may lead to withdrawal from learning and consequent feelings of disappointment and failure.

 © THE SAINSBURY CENTRE FOR MENTAL HEALTH, 2002

BOX 1 One student's experience of a named contact

"We met at the centre for an informal chat. I have always regarded that meeting as a vital link in my progression toward college life. For a start, it felt important that (the guidance worker) came to see me in my 'mental health' setting, which I valued and that she accepted me there.

"By the end (of the meeting) I had a package of information about a range of fascinating courses, a wide choice of opportunities tailored to my own interests and aspirations, a date for a follow-up discussion and arrangements for a guided tour of the college 'just to get a feel of the place'.

"The guidance worker wrote an instant summary of our discussions with a copy for each of us to keep. That was particularly useful, not only as an 'aide-memoire', but more significantly as a personal record of my aims and objectives and a tangible reminder of what I might be capable of achieving. By then I was 'hooked'." (Student).

Courses set up specifically for mental health service users

> *"If you are having a bad day and just burst into tears no one is going to ostracise you. I have also noticed how much it has brought us together outside of our prospective (day) centres in being able to share problems, generally giving us more confidence, so to speak in the outside world."* (Student)

While some people use the opportunity to return to learning as a chance to shed the mental health label and start afresh, others prefer to join a learning opportunity where their mental health label is open and acknowledged.

However, there is always the danger that courses set up for people with specific needs can either become too comfortable or they are a dead-end and consequently students never leave them. In planning such provision it is essential to ensure that the students do have the opportunity to move on to other courses, perhaps those that offer accreditation or take place in more challenging environments such as within the college itself.

The range of available courses is enormous and the most successful are where the students choose what they want learn. While not all courses lead to qualifications it is important for providers to identify the learning outcomes of every planned course.

One adult education centre set up a course in a local psychiatric hospital for patients on long-stay wards. The people on the wards chose to study the history of the hospital. The learning goals included the history of the hospital but also involved reading, writing, participating in groups, interpreting information, ordering thoughts and presenting written material.

The group produced a booklet for sale outside the hospital to help reduce the stigma about mental ill health. In addition, participating in the course helped participants to re-discover old skills and subsequently many of them became more active in the day-to-day routines of the wards. As people engaged in learning, producing ideas and creating work, nursing staff reported that they began to see them in a new and more positive light.

Learning can take place in many settings, including hospitals, day centres, and community centres or within the college and students should have a say in where they want to study. This can provide learners with stepping-stones, as their confidence grows so they move into more integrated environments. One college set up a singing course at a local day centre. When the students got used to working together in a group and with the tutor, the course was moved to a quieter annex of the college. Before long the course was held in the music department of the main building of the college and soon after that the group were performing in public.

How a course is delivered also needs to be considered. Such things as timing, group size and the skills of the tutors will have an impact on the outcomes of learning. Students should have the opportunity at the end of the course to meet with the named person again to reflect on all the things that have been achieved – attending regularly, participating and speaking in the group, getting to know new people or meeting deadlines for assignments. In this way successes can be built on and the student can progress on to other opportunities if they wish. As one student says: *"Through going to college I have acquired self-esteem, a sense of my own value in society and a personal goal to work for."*

Learning can provide structure to a day, a reason to get out of the house or a chance to make new friends. But it is also about learning new skills or re-discovering old ones, perhaps even getting qualifications that lead to employment. Learning can boost confidence and self-esteem through discovering what you can achieve and from sensing what potential you have as an individual.

The suggestions laid out here are merely common sense rather than rocket science and mainstream funding for adult and further education can provide for all these things. Adult educators will also be aware of specific monies that are available for new initiatives and projects. Further information and advice is available from The National Organisation for Adult Learning (NIACE), Skill or the Basic Skills Agency.

 © THE SAINSBURY CENTRE FOR MENTAL HEALTH, 2002

So if you would like to set up learning provision in your area, make contact with the head or principal of your local adult, community or further education provider who will be able to pass you on to the right person in their organisation.

Useful addresses

NIACE (National Organisation for Adult Learning)
21 De Montfort Street
Leicester LE1 7GE
Can also provide details of local learning and skills councils

SKILL: National Bureau for Students with Disabilities
Chapter House
18–20 Crucifix Lane
London SE1 3JW

Basic Skills Agency
7th Floor
Commonwealth House
1–19 New Oxford Street
London WC1A 1NU

Key points

- Does your local education provider have a policy on students with mental health problems? What action have they taken to combat exclusion?
- Do students with mental health problems contribute to decision making in the college through an advisory group or similar process?
- Have education staff been offered the opportunity to receive mentoring by colleagues in mental health services?
- What are the arrangements for confidentiality and disclosure of information between the learning provider and the mental health service?
- Are mental health awareness sessions offered to college staff? Are education awareness sessions offered to mental health staff?
- Has someone been identified to open up educational opportunities and provide effective guidance and support to people with mental health problems?
- Are students with mental health problems registering for mainstream courses as well as discrete 'user-only' classes?
- In the formal sessions, are people enjoying, learning and receiving accreditation? Are they joining in with the social life and activities of the college?

© THE SAINSBURY CENTRE FOR MENTAL HEALTH, 2002

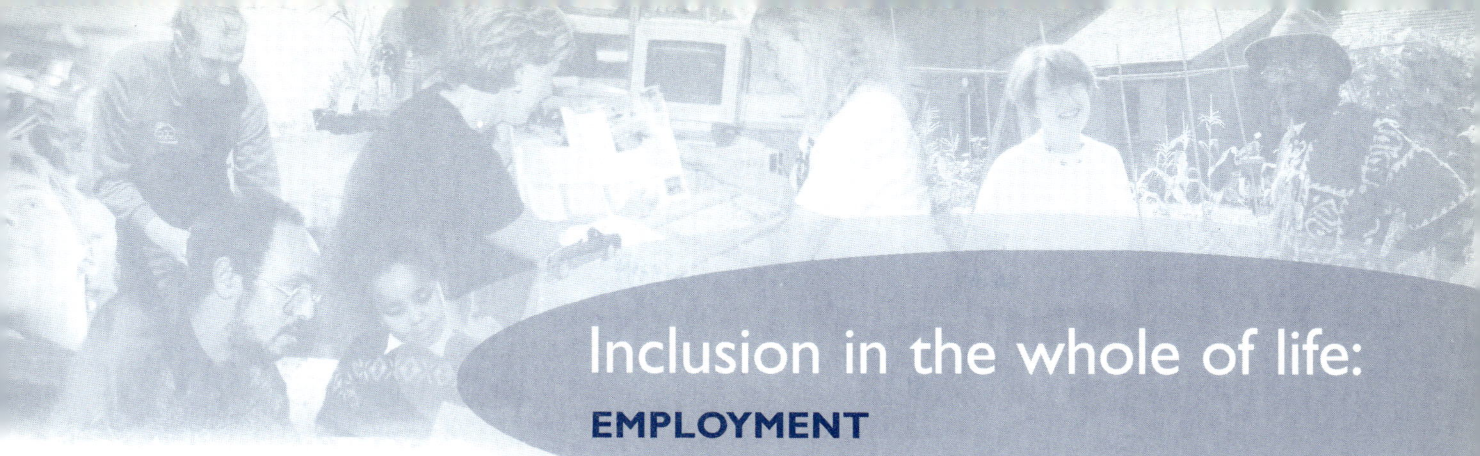

Inclusion in the whole of life: EMPLOYMENT

Justine Schneider

Social inclusion through employment is a more realistic prospect for people with severe mental health problems than ever before. There are several complementary reasons why this is so in the UK today.

Firstly, as always, there is a steady demand for paid work on the part of people with mental health problems, their carers and advocates. Secondly, there is broad legislative provision to protect the right to work of all disabled people. Thirdly, there are policy guidelines, several of which have an objective of social inclusion, that highlight the importance of employment. Fourthly, there is a growing body of practice knowledge about how to help people with mental health problems achieve employment. And, finally, there is sound evidence of the effectiveness of at least one type of employment intervention.

Once basic needs for treatment, shelter and food are met, most people want constructive activities. These allow us to use our skills, to meet people and to have a purpose to each day. Ideally, work activity is rewarded with adequate pay, so that people who obtain employment can support themselves, wholly or in part. Social interaction, having a purpose or a role in society, and the self-sufficiency that comes from gainful employment can be seen as three dimensions of social inclusion, but they are not the only indicators that can be applied.

Policy and practice

The objective of social inclusion can be seen as a theme running through a stream of social policy that provides legislation and guidelines to promote employment for all disabled people. This policy includes as its legislative foundations the *Disability Discrimination Act*, the *National Minimum Wage Act*, and the *Human Rights Act*. It finds expression in the policy guidelines laid out in the *National Service Framework for Mental Health* (Department of Health, 1999b) where the guidelines for enhanced care programmes state that consideration should be given to employment needs.

 © THE SAINSBURY CENTRE FOR MENTAL HEALTH, 2002

However, policy alone is ineffective without some technological 'know how' and the sort of experience that teaches us how best to implement guidelines. This type of practice knowledge has been gained in the past decade or more at international, national and local levels.

At the international level there have been trans-national European initiatives designed to foster innovation in the employment of disabled people, including those programmes known as Horizon, Helios and Accept. In the USA a survey (Wehman *et al.*, 1998) showed that tens of thousands of people with mental health problems are in paid employment.

The lessons learned from the experience of these individuals and the programmes and agencies that support them can be drawn upon to inform developments in the UK. At the national level, practice experience has been gained over many years from the Department of Education and Employment's supported placement scheme, which in 2001 evolved into the Workstep programme.

More recently, some of the New Deal for Disabled People pilots have provided a test bed for developing employment projects for people with mental health problems. Locally, over the years since community care for people with mental health problems has become the norm, many health trusts, local authorities and voluntary organisations have fostered employment schemes.

At present in the UK, the training and employment of disabled people, including those with severe mental health problems, also has institutional support through the Disability Rights Commission, the Social Care Institute of Excellence, the National Social Care Council, the Learning and Skills Councils and the Working Age Agencies. Joint Implementation Plans (Welfare to Work) should link the partner agencies with an interest in employment and disabilities in each local authority area.

The legislative, policy and practice knowledge and institutional structure outlined here mean that employment for people with mental health problems can be justified, promoted and protected as never before.

Of course, there are still many shortcomings. One of these is the lack of a smooth interface with the benefits system. This means that there may be little advantage in working for pay, or indeed there may be a disadvantage for some people who could lose entitlements. Another shortcoming is the fact that the technical expertise for helping people gain employment is not widespread, and does not yet form part of standard community mental health care. Thirdly, some programmes, for historical or ideological reasons, may be oriented more towards day care than employment, and the transition from one model of practice to another is often difficult to make.

 © THE SAINSBURY CENTRE FOR MENTAL HEALTH, 2002

Five models

Despite these and other difficulties, the policy and practice agenda gains impetus from the demand for occupational activities from service users and carers. Various models of employment for people with mental health problems are in operation (Pozner *et al.*, 1996; Schneider, 1998). The most common types are sheltered workshops, the transitional employment model used by clubhouses, social firms, vocational rehabilitation prior to job finding, and the individual placement and support (IPS) model of supported employment. Here, these selected models will be described briefly before we go on to consider the part they can play in increasing social inclusion for people with mental health problems.

Sheltered workshops

Sheltered workshops originated in long stay hospitals to provide constructive activities for patients. Typically, they carried out assembly work for outside contractors. With hospital closures and the development of more community-based mental health care, some workshops moved into 'open' settings, and many developed their own small enterprises doing work such as printing, furniture making and other crafts. The sheltered workshops that survive often employ older people who have spent large periods of their life in hospital and who are likely to live in specialist accommodation (Hallam and Schneider, 1999).

The worker's outputs, and the workshop's profitability are often subsidiary concerns to the therapeutic benefits of attendance at the sheltered workshop. Hence a health trust, social services department or voluntary organisation frequently underwrites the sheltered workshop.

Transitional employment programme (TEP)

This type of employment is one goal of clubhouses, which are basically structured day centres run largely by service users. The clubhouse movement, which began in the United States, trains service users and paid staff to operate within their particular ethos of participation and empowerment.

A clubhouse is likely to offer a refuge, a meeting place, a daily meal, some social activities and the opportunity to try employment through TEP. The jobs obtained in this way are technically held by the clubhouse, which is committed to filling each post with someone. If a service user doing a TEP job is unwell on a given day another service user or member of staff may have to do the job so the clubhouse fulfils its contract.

 © THE SAINSBURY CENTRE FOR MENTAL HEALTH, 2002

The jobs are normally 'entry-level', such as cleaning, gardening, catering, and clerical work. Service users are assigned to jobs for six months at a time to enable them to gain experience. The job is supposed to rotate every six months, allowing more than one person to gain experience in that post. The original post holder may move on to another TEP placement, to open employment or none. Only a small proportion of people attending a clubhouse will be on TEP at any one time, and people attending the clubhouse are not obliged to do this type of work.

Social firms

Social firms are businesses where a significant proportion of members of staff have disabilities or disadvantages in the marketplace. Every worker is paid the going rate for the job, and has equal employment rights and obligations. There were about 62 social firms operating in the UK in 1998, employing on average about six people each, of whom about two had a disability of some kind. The average turnover was £136,000 per annum (Higgins and Gianniba, 1999).

Work ranges from retail, through catering and crafts to recycling. Social firms are typical of small businesses in many ways: they can provide a very diverse range of goods and services, they come and go depending upon the conditions in the marketplace, and they are compelled to be flexible to survive.

Vocational rehabilitation

This kind of rehabilitation entails all types of preparation for work, from education and training, to assistance with job finding, applications, interview preparation and follow-up support.

Training projects may be located in further education colleges, and work placements with employers to gain experience are sometimes part of the programme. It is not clear how much vocational rehabilitation is being offered as such in the UK today and some providers of vocational rehabilitation would say that they are following the model of supported employment defined later.

Vocational rehabilitation has been unfavourably compared with the individual placement and support (IPS) model of supported employment in terms of its speed and effectiveness at obtaining paid jobs for individuals with mental health problems (Drake *et al*, 1999a, 1999b). The comparison is characterised as 'train and place' (vocational rehabilitation), versus 'place and train' (IPS).

 © THE SAINSBURY CENTRE FOR MENTAL HEALTH, 2002

However, other outcome measures need to be taken into consideration besides job tenure and earnings, such as personal development, the satisfaction of service users and long-term maintenance of employment.

Supported employment

The terms of supported employment stipulate that disabled people should have real jobs for real pay. It is defined in the recent *Policy Framework* published by the Joseph Rowntree Foundation (O'Bryan *et al.*, 2000).

Supported employment starts from the assumption that all disabled people may wish to access paid work, and that no individual or group should be seen as unemployable.

Agencies typically offer a combination of vocational profiling and helping people identify their skills and preferences. To this extent there may be considerable overlap with vocational rehabilitation as described above. Supported employment also includes: job development to find the person's preferred job through contact with employers; job analysis to find out more about the workplace, co-workers, and the support the individual might need in that environment; support to ensure that both the employee and employer receive 'just enough' back-up to achieve success, with this support continuing as long as it is needed; and career support to help people think in the longer term about career progression.

These tasks are the aspects of liaison with employers and post-placement support that distinguish IPS from most other types of vocational interventions. Some mental health agencies in the UK have successfully used supported employment preferentially to recruit people with experience of mental illness to work in mental health trusts (Perkins *et al.*, 1997).

What works?

There is strong evidence for the effectiveness of supported employment, particularly when it is compared to other models of intervention. Most of the research has taken place in the US, and it has recently been summarised in a meta-analysis for the Cochrane database (Crowther *et al.*, 2000). This establishes the reliability of earlier findings (Bond *et al.*, 1997; Drake *et al.*, 1999a, 1999b). Therefore, for agencies seeking to implement evidence-based practice in employment and mental health, supported employment should be a high priority.

 © THE SAINSBURY CENTRE FOR MENTAL HEALTH, 2002

Promoting social inclusion through work

Each of the employment models described above may be evaluated in terms of its contribution to social inclusion, which could also be defined as social interaction, having a purpose or a role in society, and self-sufficiency.

- **Sheltered workshops** clearly supply social interaction, but this is principally with other people who also have a mental health problem, and some measure of purpose, but this is usually only peripheral to the wider society, as few sheltered workshops are truly going concerns in the open market. Finally, they scarcely ever pay enough wages that permit people to come off benefits and attain self-sufficiency.
- **The TEP** enables clubhouse members who go out to work to interact with other members of society, the job offers a purpose or role, albeit it usually a humble, low-paid one, and this may permit some people to reduce their dependency on benefits. However, it is essentially temporary, so the TEP placement only offers short-term benefits.
- **Social firms**, if they survive the vicissitudes of the market, can offer financial independence to their employees and represent employment, which affords a role or purpose in life, perhaps more so as a member of a small business than in hourly-paid, low-status jobs. And there is undoubtedly a measure of social interaction amongst employees in social firms. The difficulty is that social firms cannot accommodate the tens of thousands of people with mental health problems who want to work.
- **Vocational rehabilitation** is more inclusive if it is undertaken in a non-stigmatised setting, such as a local education college, and if students with disabilities are taught alongside non-disabled students. It may offer the 'role' of student, at least temporarily, but it does not immediately permit its beneficiaries to become self-sufficient, since vocational rehabilitation is by definition simply a prelude to employment.
- **Supported employment** explicitly espouses social inclusion, and due to its principle of real jobs for real pay, supported employment is as likely as social firms to permit financial self-sufficiency, social integration, and jobs with a purpose or a role in society.

Of the models described then, social firms and supported employment most closely approximate to the ideals of social inclusion. Other models may be useful as preparatory stages for people who are recovering from severely disabling illnesses. However, a growing body of research in the US suggests that, for samples of people with severe mental health problems who themselves express a wish to work, the individual placement and support model of supported employment is more effective at obtaining open employment than other approaches. Compared to social firms, supported employment is likely to be available to more people, since it is geared towards filling vacancies in the job market, rather than the setting up of businesses, with its attendant costs and risks.

 © THE SAINSBURY CENTRE FOR MENTAL HEALTH, 2002

Conclusion

The development of models of community care, including assertive outreach and crisis intervention as required by the *National Service Framework for Mental Health*, ought therefore to entail the promotion of supported employment opportunities. While mental health teams may be unaccustomed to providing occupational inputs, they could utilise employment resources for disabled people by building links with learning skills agencies, working age agencies, workstep providers and other agencies promoting supported employment and social firms for disabled people.

Carers and service users, for their part, could ensure that mental health teams attend to the occupational needs of people on the care programme approach. From another perspective, service providers, carers and some users are employees and employers themselves. When vacant posts arise, we should all ask ourselves whether the job is one that could be done by a person with mental health problems, or how it could be adapted to be more suitable.

Key points

- Are sufficient resources available to ensure that users have access to meaningful daytime activity?
- What is the balance between day activities and employment projects?
- Do you have the right kind of employment projects?
- Do local mental health organisations employ service users in sufficient numbers and in the right jobs?

 © THE SAINSBURY CENTRE FOR MENTAL HEALTH, 2002

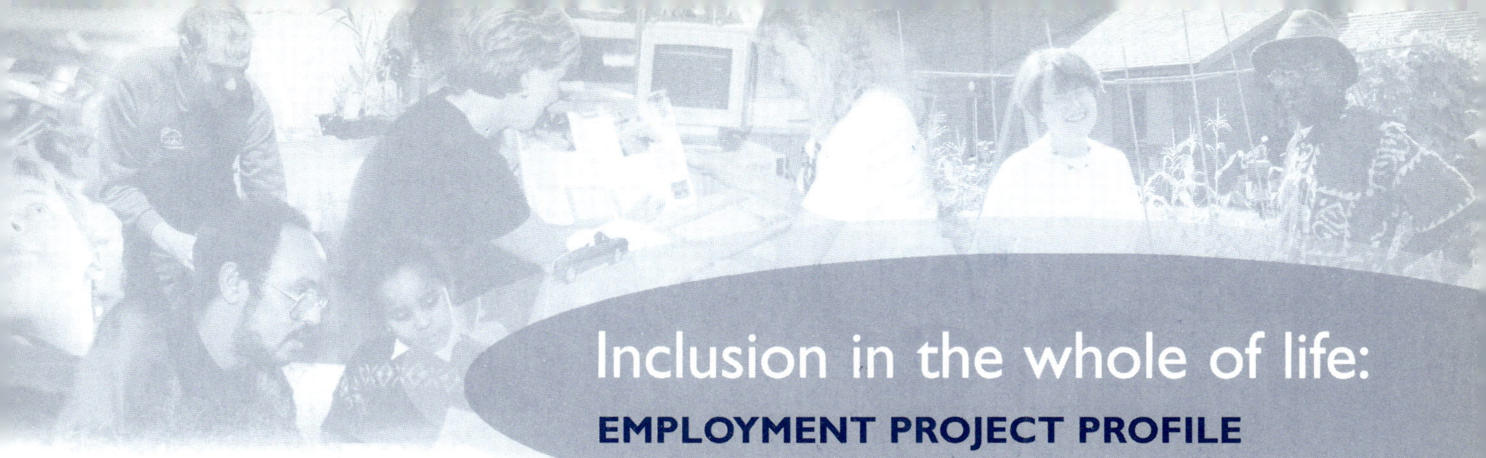

Inclusion in the whole of life:
EMPLOYMENT PROJECT PROFILE

Penny Robertson, Louise Knox and
K. Gilyead, Pentreath Industries Ltd

Pentreath Industries is a registered charity providing 'gateways to employment for people with or recovering from mental ill health in Cornwall'.

Since its foundation in 1990, Pentreath has constantly challenged the assumption that those who have undergone the trauma of a psychiatric illness will still retain its residual reminders and are capable of little more than employment at a basic level. Pentreath has evidence that when provided with suitable support and skills update, the great majority of its clients are capable of re-entering employment at a variety of levels of responsibility.

Pentreath has identified the essential requirements of employers, monitored changes over time and responded by providing training opportunities for service users in numeracy, literacy, and communication and information technology. This has encouraged the development of new skills. In addition, the up-skills and re-skills needed by many of our clients are simply the basic industrial competencies of working as a member of a team, accepting responsibility for the quality of one's work, accepting instruction or criticism and punctuality and regular attendance. These skills are often submerged or damaged by the 'numbing' experience of psychosis.

Funding is via a range of sources including Cornwall Healthcare NHS Trust, the European Social Fund, the Employment Service via the New Deal provision, National Lotteries Charity Board, Cornwall College, grant giving trusts, and sale of products and services. A team of 76 staff provided long-term support for 598 service users in 2000 that were referred from community mental health teams. Since 1996 an average of 30 people have moved from Pentreath into full-time waged employment each year.

All areas of service delivery are underpinned by the need to create the environment and opportunity for people to work, live, socialise and contribute as full citizens in their community. To deliver these ambitions the company concentrates on four main areas of service delivery:

- training;
- employment placement advice;

 © THE SAINSBURY CENTRE FOR MENTAL HEALTH, 2002

- social firm development;
- raising awareness of mental health issues.

While this list has been constructed to show how an individual might progress from training to placement in open employment or into a social firm, and finally to impact the attitudes of the wider community (see **box 1**), it could easily have been reversed to suggest that public awareness opens the door to opportunities for individuals. All these elements are interdependent.

BOX 1 One user's experience of training

"Pentreath is probably the most positive thing that I have been offered as a person with a mental illness. I have been attending for six months and it has made a great difference to me.

"Because of my illness and because of people's attitude to my illness, I had lost all confidence in my ability to work and interact socially. It is wonderful to be treated with respect and understanding by people who 'know' and to be able to interact with both staff and other clients as an individual. It is also very important to me to be making a useful contribution.

"Pentreath is providing me with the opportunity to find out what strengths I have and to develop them within a safe environment. It also enables me to recognise my limitations and to seek and experiment with healthy strategies for coping with them. This is helping me to put myself and my illness into perspective, which is helping to build my confidence, enabling me to function more efficiently, and hopefully improving my prospects.

"My only complaint is that Pentreath is not more accessible; I do a round trip of about eighty-two miles a day." (K. Gilyead)

Pentreath aims to offer a range of training opportunities to improve employability of people with or recovering from mental ill health. In addition to courses provided by our trainers, who are all professionally qualified in their training area, a close relationship with Cornwall College of Further Education has enabled the development of a range of courses on topics including computer skills and internet access, environmental conservation, health and safety in the workplace, financial management, numeracy and communication skills.

Franchising has enabled educational services to be offered at Pentreath for people who feel unable to access courses at college, as well as enriching the supply of technical support and expertise. In addition, some courses at college are provided for Pentreath trainees only, with both the college and Pentreath providing a member of staff.

Individual coaching, transport and reduced college fees assist some people to engage. An individual action plan helps to build confidence and self-esteem so that students transfer from Pentreath to mainstream settings including public transport, education, community facilities and employment (see **box 2**). An annual presentation event offers an opportunity for trainees to invite guests to celebrate the achievement of nationally accredited qualifications as well as enjoying dinner and a disco.

As well as the specific courses leading to qualifications, training is offered to service users to support their participation in the activities of Pentreath itself, such as membership of the stakeholders group.

BOX 2 A user's experience of employment placement advice

"Although very nervous of the project, I took advice from my social worker and decided to work with Pentreath. My first contact with Pentreath was with an employment placement advisor (EPA) who did an initial interview. I was very tentative at this stage with low self-esteem and confidence. We said that a good option would be to find a work placement, which allowed me to gradually overcome these problems. With an EPA fully supporting me in this work placement I was able to increase my confidence.

"After a period of time I felt I was able to try out something new. I tried computers. I soon discovered an ability to operate computers; this came as a major surprise. I could now look in other areas of work. This changed my plans completely. I took up a work placement with a local council as a data input clerk. I have now changed my whole outlook on job prospects, with further training and work experience, new opportunities are open to me."

Sixteen EPAs on the staff of Pentreath arrange work experience and support to individuals wishing to return to work. They undertake vocational assessment, identify aspirations and work with the person to create a route to achieving these goals.

 © THE SAINSBURY CENTRE FOR MENTAL HEALTH, 2002

Where necessary, training is located to support the person to realise his or her aspirations. The EPA has a duty to ensure that employers do not exploit individuals and their specialism is in providing support, motivation and information for employers and potential employees.

While work experience only attracts therapeutic payments it has provided the opportunity for people to build skills, experience and social networks, and 85% of the salaried jobs obtained have been as a direct result of work experience.

In general, our experience with employers has been very positive. By working individually we have highlighted how common mental illness is and how much hidden support employers can and do give. In addition, co-workers have responded positively towards people with a mental health problem in the workplace.

Social firm development

Social firms offer paid employment opportunities within smaller, community-based commercial enterprises that aim to pay market-level wages and have integrated workforces – people with and without mental health issues working alongside each other (see **box 3**). The following steps can help create a social firm:

- Appoint a motivating project leader who is committed to democratic approaches.
- Form a management group of people who want to work in the social firm, while discouraging clinical involvement in the management group.
- Invest time in team building by visiting and learning from other social firms.
- Carry out market research – with training and good preparation it can be a lot of fun and help with the development of the new business.
- Write a business plan for the social firm.
- Encourage entrepreneurship. Developing a new business is risky and this needs to be acknowledged. Promote an adaptable, 'no blame' culture.
- Recruit people from the local business community and economic development officers to form a business advisory group to provide expert advice.
- Develop an ethos of working together to support both staff members and business flexibility.
- Develop businesses that require a range of skill sets, providing work for all on both good days and days when concentration may not be so good.
- Foster ambition.

 © THE SAINSBURY CENTRE FOR MENTAL HEALTH, 2002

BOX 3 A user's experience of the 'real world' of work

"The opportunity at Lyonesse Trading Places (LTP) came at just the right time for me. I wanted to get back into work and had looked at some jobs, but lacked the confidence to make the final step. What I needed was more confidence, more self-esteem. That's what I was able to get at LTP. The chance to work in a friendly environment with consideration for the fact that I'd been ill, and no pressure, was just what I needed.

"Doing useful, interesting work is an important thing. It's nice to work on a product like Cornish World magazine, that's sold in the real world. Using computers is good too, a chance to learn 'up to the minute' and useful skills, but at your own pace until you grow in confidence.

"Also at LTP you have the chance to try out different things. If you prefer working outside there's the Greenscape gardening project, or perhaps Pedals, the bike hire and repair company. I've recently been involved in the latest project – neat document management (archiving documents onto computer disk using the latest software). Different jobs suit different people, or if you like you can split your time between various things.

"LTP has certainly been a godsend for me. I'm very glad that the opportunity came along when it did."

Charles* at LTP Penzance (* name changed at the request of the author).

Pentreath Industries' diverse range of emerging social firms includes:

- Heaven Scent, a wholesale nursery, which sells plants to the prestigious Eden Project and contributed to the college display at the Chelsea Flower Show.
- *Cornish World* magazine, a glossy subscriber magazine produced for 'lovers of Cornwall at home and abroad'. Subscribers are not aware that it is part of a mental health social firm. As sales improve the management committee will decide whether they wish to publicise their history of mental illness.
- Pedals, a cycle hire and bike renovation business located on the Cornish cycle way.
- Trevaylor Hotel.

At Pentreath we have found that social firms offer a small number of people an exciting opportunity to create sustainable employment for themselves. They are not suitable for everyone and some people find democratic working methods frustrating and prefer a more autocratic environment.

 © THE SAINSBURY CENTRE FOR MENTAL HEALTH, 2002

While considerable investment is needed in team building and planning, this is critical in ensuring shared ownership of the project and achieving a healthy balance between meeting business goals and supporting individual staff members. Staff members who have a commitment to the business and to their work colleagues find it is an effective environment for building confidence and skills, developing friends and gaining real wages for real work.

Raising awareness of mental health issues

A key part of the mission of Pentreath industries is to promote mental health and develop a positive community response. The aim is to raise awareness of the impact and prevalence of mental ill health in the locality, while practically demonstrating the way in which barriers can be lowered to enable all citizens to achieve their ambitions of recovery, inclusion and contribution to their locality. In order to do this, we have forged links with a wide variety of agencies (see **box 4**).

BOX 4 Linked agencies

- Chamber of Commerce
- Social Firms UK and Social Firms Southwest
- Regional Development Agency
- Southern Association for Voluntary Action Groups for Europe
- National Council for Voluntary Organisations
- Cornwall Voluntary Sector Forum
- Citizens Advice Bureaux
- Health Action Zone
- Employment Service Disability Employment Advisors
- New Deal Personal Advisors
- Devon and Cornwall Learning and Skills Council
- Community Action Team
- Employment Action Team
- Economic Regeneration Boards
- Government Office Southwest
- European Office in Brussels
- Co-operative Movement
- Cornwall Business Club
- DSS Benefits Agency
- Cornwall Healthcare NHS Trust
- Cornwall and Isles of Scilly Health Authority
- Primary Care Groups/Trusts
- Link into Learning
- Cornwall College

© THE SAINSBURY CENTRE FOR MENTAL HEALTH, 2002

A stakeholder group that includes service users, funders, employers and representatives of key agencies guides the way in which Pentreath is run.

The group's work has led to the introduction of agreements with employers that specify responsibilities for work experience placements, new opportunities for people previously excluded from employment due to their challenging mental health needs, and improved liaison with the Benefits Agency.

Promoting a positive image requires action at many levels, from negotiation with public sector agencies to daily work patterns. For example, a recent survey demonstrated the high value placed on everyone wearing the same uniform at Pentreath – it is smart, provides protection and challenges perceptions, as visitors cannot distinguish between staff and trainees. Finally, people from the business community sit on the board of management at Pentreath, and have provided specialist assistance.

Conclusion

It is vital to involve all stakeholders to ensure that services are developed that are appropriate to the needs of participants and these partnerships provide a chance to share resources, expertise and funding. We provide a full range of services so that participants can enjoy the full range of training and employment choice available in the wider community so that personal potential can be realised.

Key points

At Pentreath...

- A wide variety of partners and funding sources have been harnessed, bringing health, education and employment agencies to the same table.
- The organisation listens to service user accounts of mental health problems, the importance of work and what has been helpful.
- Education opportunities have been developed through direct provision and franchising, on and off site, in discrete classes and through mainstream registration.
- Individual action plans focus on training and work.
- A number of social firms have been developed through concentrating the 'start-up' expertise in the same organisation.

 © THE SAINSBURY CENTRE FOR MENTAL HEALTH, 2002

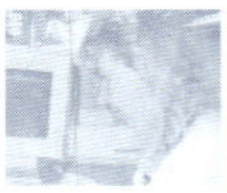

Case Study

Jason was referred to the clubhouse by his psychiatrist in 1995. He was a pleasant, friendly young man of 20 diagnosed as having schizophrenia but who had failed to come to terms with his mental illness and the medication he had to take. He had suffered bullying at school and was rather withdrawn at home.

Jason lived with his brother, sister and parents who, though obviously caring and concerned, seemed to have too much control of his life. A parent (usually the father) went with Jason to appointments with the psychiatrist and, it seems, did most of the talking. There were also family arguments from time to time and some of these were around Jason's lack of money management.

At the beginning, although Jason was happy to come to the clubhouse, he did not easily attach to any of the work units or relate particularly to any other members. He was encouraged to come in on regular days and take on specific tasks as well as taking ownership of his health situation, being aware of signs of relapse and the action he needed to take.

An essential part of the clubhouse model is the Transitional Employment Programme (TEP) that offers part-time temporary placements at the going rate of pay. There is a considerable amount of support available from clubhouse staff, as well as on the job training.

In the summer of 1996, Jason was approached to see if he was interested in taking up a placement at Marks & Spencer Plc that would shortly become available. This entailed working on the shop floor for just three hours per week, putting out new stock, tidying racks of garments and answering customers' queries as they arose. Jason was keen to take this up although there were a few concerns about his timekeeping and his personal presentation as, apart from working for a food store for three months, he had not had a 'proper' job before. He quickly settled into the job and obviously enjoyed it.

By the end of the nine-month placement, Jason had proved to be a good and willing worker and he was anxious to continue. He let the personnel office know he was seeking work and was fortunate that there was a part time vacancy for twelve hours per week available. He successfully applied for this and started working independently for Marks & Spencer in July 1997 while continuing to attend goal setting reviews at the clubhouse.

By the end of 2000 he was working 28 hours per week with occasional extra work during the holiday period. Jason is a very well respected member of Marks & Spencer's staff team. He has received two customer care awards and has an excellent rapport with customers. The clubhouse continues to have a good working relationship with Marks & Spencer.

© THE SAINSBURY CENTRE FOR MENTAL HEALTH, 2002

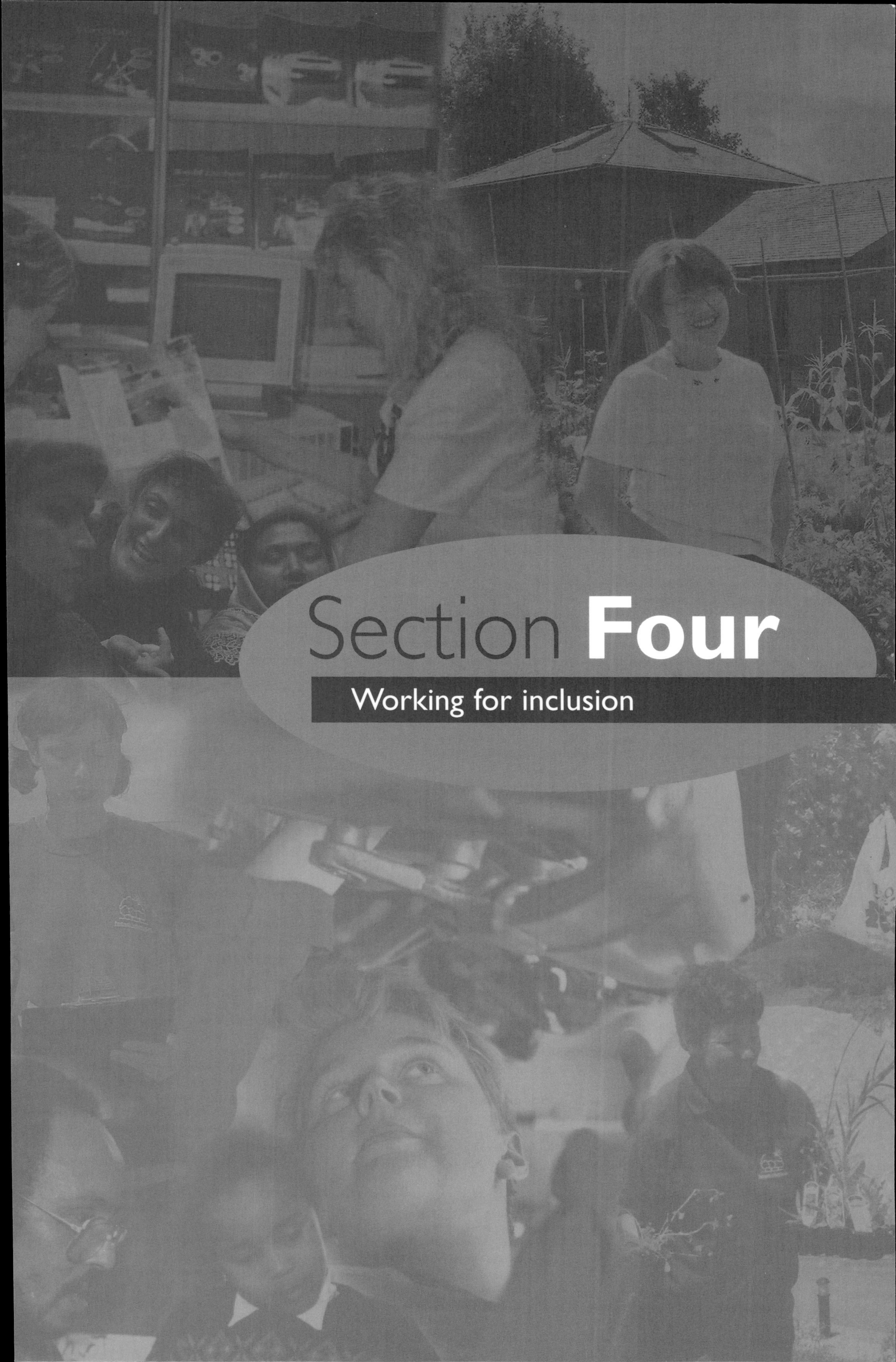

Section **Four**

Working for inclusion

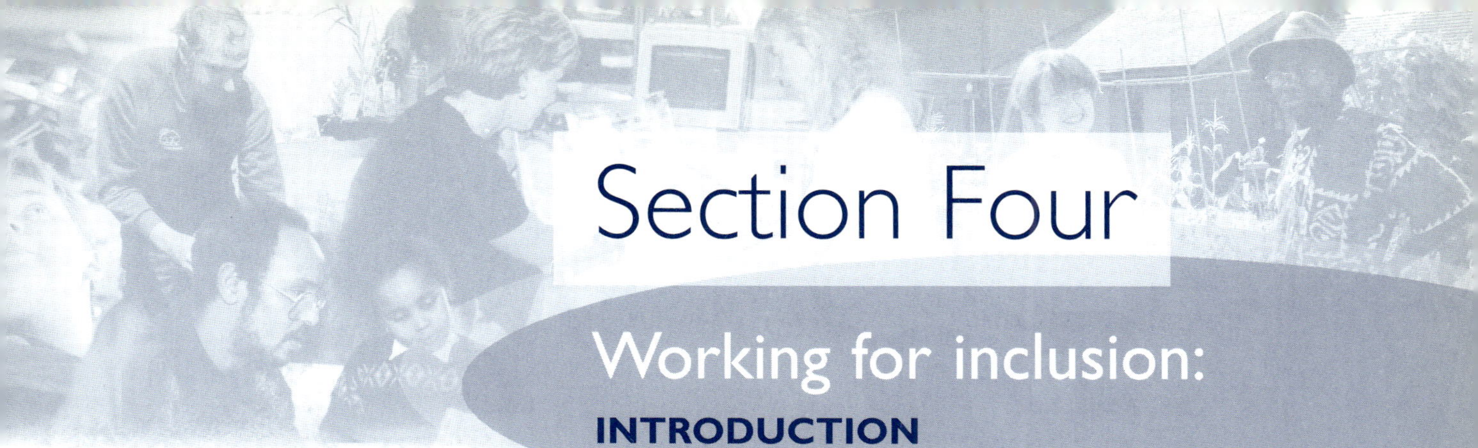

Section Four

Working for inclusion: INTRODUCTION

Peter Bates

In his book on community-based support for people with mental health problems, Paul Carling (1995) sets out his expectation that people look to their personal resources before seeking formal assistance from mental health services.

Personal coping strategies, combined with informal support from family and friends proves to be the first line of defence against distress. Personal coping strategies form one area that is targeted by mental health promotion work, while initiatives to promote social inclusion help people to maintain positive social roles and receive support from friends and colleagues.

This section of the book shows how mental health services can contribute to social inclusion. Traditional mental health services have often severed the connection between service users and their informal community, either by neglect or through blaming. We show that mental health services can be re-designed to promote community membership and participation, for the web of friendships, roles and identities that form community is intrinsic to recovery.

The contributions in this section broadly follow a career through the service system, starting with primary care, where most people receive initial help with mental health problems. David Morris and Sara Weech describe the work that they carried out with primary care groups and trusts. This study generated a set of indicators that can be used by these primary care organisations to benchmark their progress in developing inclusive mental health services. While some of these factors appear to be necessary rather than sufficient to create inclusive opportunities, they form a valuable starting point for agencies willing to listen to the challenge that each indicator might pose.

Anna Barnes and Toni Wilkinson report on their progress in Hastings and St Leonard's Primary Care Trust. This work is distinctive in two ways. Firstly, it highlights how new agencies can start with a high degree of service user involvement in the planning process, rather than needing to build up to this over an extended time, as some longer-standing organisations have done. Secondly, the primary care trust has built some significant alliances with partners in the education, crime and disorder and regeneration agencies, showing that top-level collaboration is a key requirement for delivering inclusive opportunities at the grass roots.

While many people can be supported in a primary care setting, others need specialist assistance and the next article addresses the issues around early intervention. Ruth Marriott shows that reaching young people with psychosis can significantly improve their life chances and describes a service that places specialist advice and support within a non-stigmatising setting.

Indeed, the use of generic community settings for mental health care is a simple and effective means of promoting inclusion. While outpatient clinics have been provided in GP surgeries since the 1960s, it would appear that the inconvenience to staff of using generic settings may have overshadowed the benefits to service users. As a result mental health service managers have often continued to invest capital in property rather than revenue in rental charges. Ruth Marriott's article gives a vivid example of the potential advantages of lowering the barriers between the mental health services and neighbouring providers.

Despite the best efforts of primary care and community staff using early intervention approaches, some individuals spend time on the acute psychiatric ward. Julie Repper and Rachel Perkins explain how this can be valuable time out from the pressures of specific roles and relationships but can also be used positively to retain or rebuild inclusive opportunities. This immensely practical article cuts through the workload pressures that can threaten to engulf staff and reminds everyone of the real needs of the individual and his or her family and friends. Inclusion is not an extra to be added on in a few spare minutes of the day, but a defining characteristic of the acute setting.

Finally, Andrew Gibb describes some work with people who have spent a long time in contact with psychiatric services. *Mainstream* runs almost no groups itself, but offers daytime opportunities in ordinary community settings alongside other citizens. Staff called 'bridge-builders' expand the capacity of communities to welcome people with mental health problems, working in education, employment and volunteering, in arts, faith and sports communities.

Careful attention is paid to the hopes and dreams of each person, and then support is tailored to their preference and the environment and community they wish to join. This project is distinctive in its interest in the whole sweep of community life, rather than just employment or education, and for the person-centred approach to providing support that is demonstrated by the team.

 © THE SAINSBURY CENTRE FOR MENTAL HEALTH, 2002

This section, like others in the publication is incomplete. Staff from regional secure units and high security hospitals have been reflecting on how they might promote social inclusion in the way that they work with individuals. Forensic and addiction services are often concerned about how to assist service users in substituting a new community for the friendship circle that has sustained their destructive behaviour, and so are negotiating a particularly complex route towards social inclusion.

Some inclusive work with children has been well-documented (Newton and Wilson, 1999) but less progress has been made on supporting young people with psychiatric difficulties in mainstream education and social settings. While a start has been made in applying inclusive thinking to services for older people with a learning disability (Janicki and Ansello, 2000; Walker and Walker, 1998), there is a great deal yet to do in examining the application of inclusive thinking to psychogeriatric services. Finally, inclusive approaches might offer a great deal to people who have a learning disability in addition to mental health problems.

 © THE SAINSBURY CENTRE FOR MENTAL HEALTH, 2002

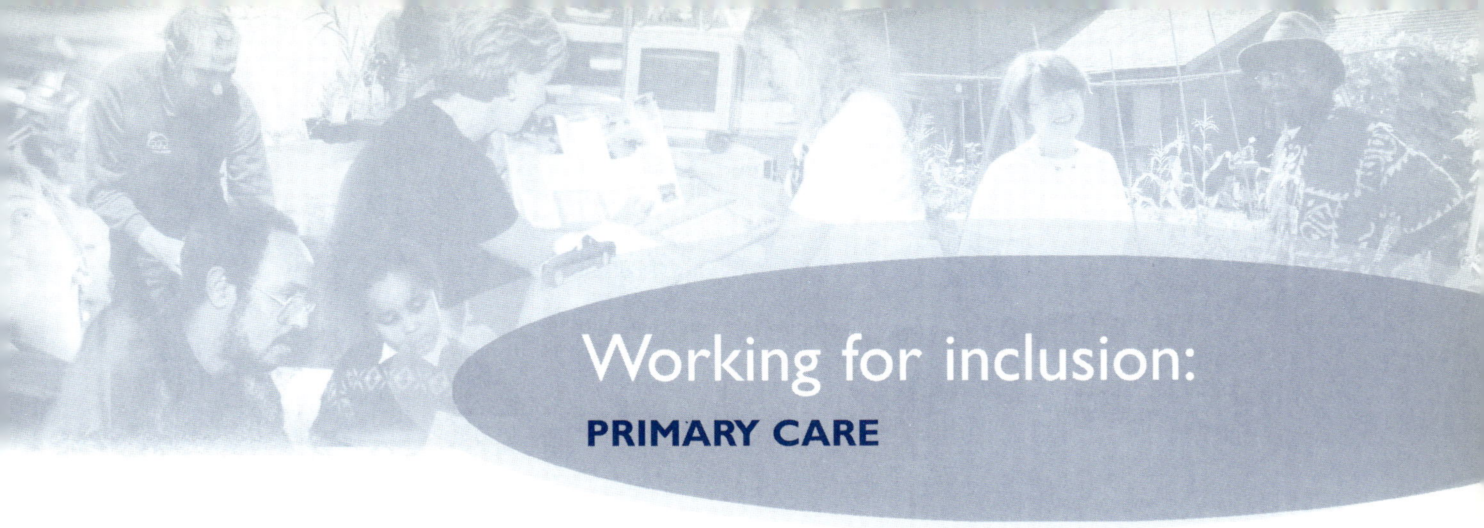

Working for inclusion:
PRIMARY CARE

David Morris and Sara Weech

One of the projects that makes up the Citizenship and Community Programme at the Sainsbury Centre for Mental Health investigated primary care organisations and their stance on social inclusion.

This project was developed by the NHS South East Regional Office in collaboration with the National Primary Care Research and Development Centre in Manchester in response to three major developments in social and healthcare policy:

- The *National Service Framework for Mental Health (NSF)* (Department of Health, 1999b).
- The formation of primary care organisations as local accountable health organisations responsible for commissioning and providing community care to a small population group.
- The social inclusion agenda that provides an opportunity to influence mental health services and enhance the capacity of communities to respond to those with mental health needs.

Linked to other work on the NSF and social inclusion, the project was based on the premise that primary care organisations should play a central role in promotion of social inclusion and equitable service provision.

The project developed and validated a set of ten indicators for primary care organisations against which their progress in implementing the NSF and promoting social inclusion could be tracked and assessed (see **box 1**). The participating primary care organisations considered that achieving a good score on the following ten elements means that the organisation will be promoting social inclusion and citizenship for people with mental health problems.

 © THE SAINSBURY CENTRE FOR MENTAL HEALTH, 2002

Social inclusion through primary care

BOX 1 An assessment framework

To what extent does the primary care group or trust:

- Understand the health needs of its local population?
- Have an agreed vision for meeting the mental health needs of its population?
- Know what social and community resources are available to its population (including health and social care provision and other resources)?
- Work within clear and agreed partnership arrangements with key organisations and groups external to the health service?
- Have an established system to collect and disseminate information about services available to people with mental health problems (including information about specialist provision and non-mental health resources)?
- Have in place measures to ensure equitable distribution of primary care based mental health services?
- Have a system in place to ensure all people with severe and enduring mental illness are known and have access to primary care services?
- Have a strategy in place to identify and meet the mental health training needs of primary care staff?
- Have an effective mental health commissioning structure in place?
- Participate in strategic service planning and implementation of the National Service Framework for Mental Health?

Findings from the work included

- The indicators were accepted as appropriate and useful targets, although it was acknowledged that significant time would be required to reach all the targets.
- Leadership is critical to ensuring that the primary care organisations make a difference in terms of community development and mental health services.
- Leadership needs to be supported to ensure that innovations become mainstream over time.

© THE SAINSBURY CENTRE FOR MENTAL HEALTH, 2002

- Social inclusion is closely linked with health promotion. Primary care and mental health services need help to develop and combine health promotion and social inclusion approaches to assist in the recovery of people with mental health problems.
- More work is needed to uncover the evidence-base for working on the social inclusion agenda.
- Primary care organisations do not currently have access to organisational development or training to support the social inclusion agenda.
- Mental health services have not traditionally demonstrated an ability to develop community capacity and promote recovery. Primary care trusts have both the opportunity and the mandate to contribute to social inclusion and community development.
- Primary care organisations that are free from the immediate demand to manage changes in the specialist mental health services are able to develop innovative community resources.
- All the participating primary care organisations saw a future when community capacity was developed, there was equity of provision, and people with mental health problems were not socially excluded but supported in the community. However, there was no shared approach to achieving this desirable future.

The project is now a key project within the Sainsbury Centre for Mental Health's Citizenship and Community Programme.

 © THE SAINSBURY CENTRE FOR MENTAL HEALTH, 2002

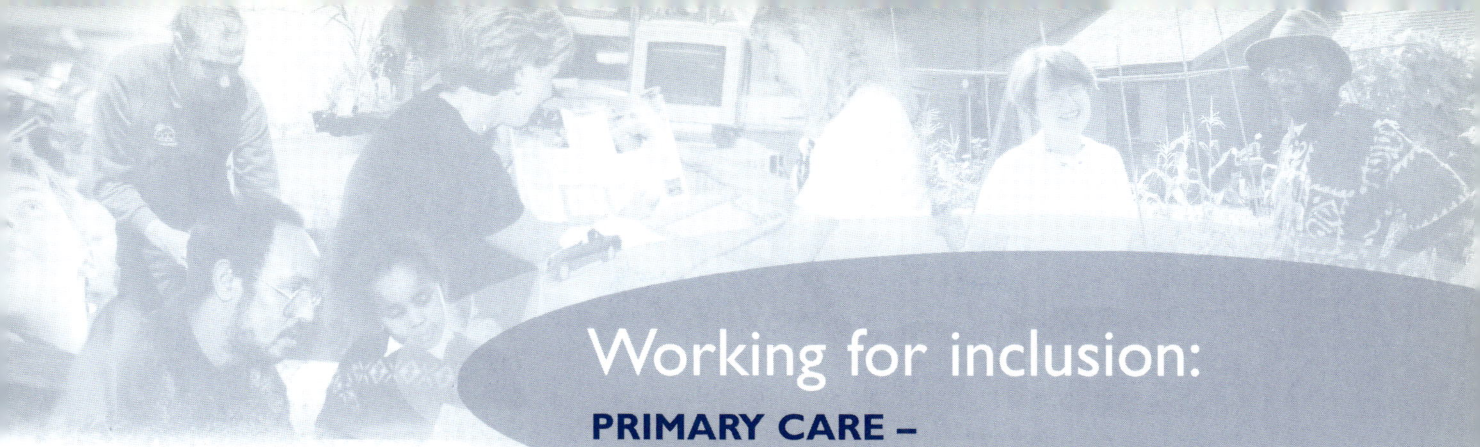

Working for inclusion:

PRIMARY CARE – A COLLABORATIVE APPROACH

Anna Barnes and Toni Wilkinson

This article describes the approach taken by Hastings and St Leonard's former Primary Care Group (now Primary Care Trust) in setting the framework for improving local mental health services in collaboration with Hastings and Rother NHS Trust.

The rationale for change and the structures that were agreed will be outlined, as will the changes in services that resulted. There will also be a general discussion about the involvement of service users and regeneration agencies in this process. Finally, the article describes how this process succeeded in putting mental health centre stage in the process of regeneration, which has resulted in greater social inclusion for the people involved.

Policy context

The NHS National Plan (Department of Health, 2000) continues the policy guidance of the past ten years in recommending that service users should be able to influence the way services are designed and delivered. The recent emphasis on social inclusion cites mental health service users as being excluded from full participation in society because of the multiple disadvantages they face such as poverty, unemployment, poor housing and social isolation (Sainsbury Centre for Mental Health, 2000). However participation is doubly difficult for mental health service users because of the following factors:

- **Discrimination:** Mental health service users are routinely ignored because of their illness. A fallacy exists that because people with psychosis sometimes suffer from delusions and hallucinations this automatically prevents them from holding rational views of the services they receive.
- **Stigma:** Some mental health service users are reluctant to identify themselves publicly as users of services and therefore do not always wish to take the opportunity to become involved in service planning.

 © THE SAINSBURY CENTRE FOR MENTAL HEALTH, 2002

- **Disadvantage:** Participating in planning often requires service users to attend committee meetings that have quite formal rules and procedures. Access to these structures is easier for people with self-confidence and a good level of education. People from disadvantaged backgrounds such as childhood abuse and the associated lower levels of education are more likely to suffer from mental illness and this is often a barrier to participation. (Pilgrim and Rogers, 1999).

Therefore, although the need to involve service users in planning services is pressing, the nature of social exclusion makes it difficult for them to become involved.

Local context

Despite the surrounding rural catchment area and scenic position on the south coast, Hastings suffers from serious urban deprivation: years of under-investment and the decline of local manufacturing and tourism industries has left the town with many problems. There is also some evidence that people with mental health and drug problems drift into the town, attracted by the availability of low cost housing and the relatively youthful population.

As a result, Hastings scores highly on both the Mental Illness Needs Index and on the Jarman index of urban deprivation. It was widely agreed that urgent action was needed to meet the needs of local people with mental health and substance misuse problems and in 1999 the local primary care group (PCG) developed a plan in collaboration with the local health trust.

The change agenda facing services was enormous. A new psychiatric unit had just been built that reduced the number of available inpatient psychiatric beds, community-based services were poorly developed and there was a lack of multi–agency consensus about the direction services should take. In addition, the community care planning structures had been centralised at county level and there was no appropriate multi-agency vehicle for decision making or debate.

The chief executive of the PCG and the director of mental health services of the trust decided to set up two multi-agency forums. These two groups were called the Mental Health Action Group (MHAG) and the Substance Misuse Action Group (SMAG). The membership grew over time as specific issues required attention (see **box 1**). Each group now has a mailing list of fifty people. It is the first time that representatives from the following agencies have met on a regular basis.

 © THE SAINSBURY CENTRE FOR MENTAL HEALTH, 2002

BOX 1 Group members

- carers
- education officers
- GPs
- health authority commissioners
- housing
- managers of the primary care and NHS trusts
- nurses
- police
- psychiatrists
- psychologists
- service users
- social services
- voluntary sector providers

With such a diverse mix of agencies, seeking consensus is not easy, so both forums operate within a framework of agreed terms of reference with an action plan.

Mechanisms for participation

As has been already identified, setting up a committee does not automatically enable people to participate. Mental health service users have found a range of ways to participate in the MHAG as follows:

- Their two chosen representatives attend meetings. One was a carer representative on the community health council, while the other is the user involvement development worker for Focus, a network of service users.
- The chair of the mental health action group (the chief executive of the primary care group) attends Focus and reports on a regular basis. Other members of the MHAG also regularly attend Focus meetings in connection with specific issues, and these debates are then reported back to the group as a whole. Focus group members have chosen this mechanism rather than attendance themselves at the MHAG.
- All group members are entitled to claim expenses for their participation.

These mechanisms mean that specific actions are agreed with Focus, and they are consulted about the issues that are discussed at the MHAG, while their participation has been adapted to suit the differing levels of ability and commitment within the group. By not attending the MHAG the users feel more in control of the agenda than by sending one user representative. They perhaps feel safer in greater numbers as approximately twenty members attend Focus as opposed to one user amongst a committee of 20 or 30 at the MHAG.

 © THE SAINSBURY CENTRE FOR MENTAL HEALTH, 2002

Relationship to commissioning

The groups are by necessity cumbersome, as all the agencies represented are separately accountable, and have different strategies and responsibilities. However, both groups have now agreed to act as local reference groups for both the drug action team (accountable to the National Treatment Agency) and the local implementation team for the *National Service Framework for Mental Health* (accountable to South Thames Regional Health Authority).

The chief executive of the PCG also sits on the Responsible Authorities Partnership that has formulated a crime reduction strategy, and the Education Action Zone. She is also the health theme leader for the Single Regeneration Budget. These wide-ranging connections enable work to be co-ordinated on crosscutting themes, for example reducing crime by increasing drug treatment services.

A firm commitment from members of the group to take action about the specific issues that are raised has made significant progress possible. Traditionally, mental health has been seen as purely a health issue, despite the clear relationship with poverty and disadvantage. This may be a legacy of the asylum system when mental health represented 'otherness' (Foucault, 1965). Therefore attempts to link mental health with regeneration, community safety, and education are laudable, although currently these links rest mainly with one person.

It is hoped that local work on Standard One of the *National Service Framework for Mental Health (NSF)*, which has started to address issues like access to education, transport and leisure opportunities will strengthen these links. Focus has been heavily involved in this work with the MHAG in its role as the local implementation team for the NSF.

The planning structures are bureaucratic but it means that the groups have a direct relationship to commissioning and can influence decisions that are made with regard to resource allocation. The relationship of service users to commissioning has thus become very direct, as the chief executive must give account to Focus for decisions made.

There have been some examples of service changes that have been challenged through this alliance between the chief executive and the users: notably the decision to shut day services as part of the NHS cost improvement programme. Managers in the NHS trust were forced to reverse this unpopular decision after discussion at the MHAG. This followed consultation and lobbying from the user group to the chief executive of the primary care group. The day service now has been given a clear commitment that it will not now be subject to cost cutting exercises. Both staff and users welcomed this.

 © THE SAINSBURY CENTRE FOR MENTAL HEALTH, 2002

Key achievements

The two action groups have been meeting monthly for two years now. At times the structure of going over agreed actions and agreeing priorities for expenditure has been complex and bureaucratic rather than productive. The sheer number of different agencies in the room sometimes means that debates have to start by explaining basic facts to ensure that everyone has the same level of understanding of the issues. This takes time. However, the achievements have been significant and a few are briefly described below:

Mental health training events

- The primary care trust funded a day conference on recovery. Service users led the day that was facilitated by Rachel Perkins with speakers from all key agencies in mental health. Eighty people attended and workshops also included aromatherapy and massage as requested by service users, as well as sessions on medication.
- A second event was led by the mental health promotion charity, **mentality**. It looked at how to develop a separate action plan to maintain and improve health rather than treat illness, and how to develop links with local employers and colleges.

Responding to crises

- Taking people off the streets into a police station under section 136 of the *Mental Health Act 1983* is stigmatising and potentially dangerous for people already vulnerable because of mental health problems. There was a proposal to establish an alternative place of safety in a separate small assessment ward adjacent to the psychiatric hospital. People with both drug and mental health problems could be assessed here instead of at the police station. The MHAG, partly due to the participation of the police in these meetings, has agreed this as a priority.
- The group lobbied for better conditions for people in the psychiatric unit, particularly for the garden to be made safer, so acutely ill people could go out.

Services

- **Mental health services directory:** This popular publication has been re-issued, using a very broad definition of good health, which links into the work on Standard One of the NSF.
- The users felt that the threats posed to day services throughout the life of the MHAG were unacceptable. They used their influence to lobby the chair to review and reverse these cuts.

 © THE SAINSBURY CENTRE FOR MENTAL HEALTH, 2002

- **One Stop Shop:** This new concept in health care has been taken up enthusiastically by Focus who would like to see this linked to mental health service provision.
- **A new multi-agency resource centre:** Regeneration funds have now been allocated to Hastings Mind to purchase a property for users as a resource centre and day centre. Before the MHAG was set up, Hastings Mind had been seeking funds for five years, occupying temporary premises and had been asked to leave them as soon as possible. Making links with regeneration officers through the two action groups proved the key to accessing funds.

Substance misuse

For five years the local trust had been advocating for an additional medical post to meet the needs of the growing population with opiate and benzodiazepine addiction. The combined commitment of the Substance Misuse Action Group (SMAG) members meant that these funds have now been found.

Dual diagnosis training programme

A multi-agency training programme was designed (at no cost) following an audit of dual diagnosis of mental illness and substance misuse that showed a 25% co-morbidity rate.

Crime and disorder initiatives

Social inclusion demands that people with addiction or other health problems should be offered the opportunity to participate in treatment programmes rather than just being swept off the streets and into custody. The SMAG decided to spend some new money available through the *NHS Plan* (Department of Health, 2000) on treatment places in order to reduce drug related crime. This has only been possible because inter-agency agreement has been reached through this forum. A similar initiative is being targeted at people who are under 18 with criminal behaviour that is caused by substance misuse. Key links have been made with the Education Action Zone.

Discussions with Focus, a network of service users

Focus members explained that they preferred to request the attendance of commissioners at their own meetings where they felt more in control, rather than attend large meetings that might feel intimidating. However, several members said that they had relied on one member of Focus to attend the action groups on their behalf, but that person had been ill and unable to attend for some time. This was seen as a weakness and several members felt they were now confident enough to attend in their own right, and would do so in future.

 © THE SAINSBURY CENTRE FOR MENTAL HEALTH, 2002

There was some concern that minutes did not always express user views, and that the agendas were preset beforehand. Once again the group felt that they wanted to change this, and have a hand in setting agendas, particularly around resource allocation. One member also queried the chief executive's accountability to them. As someone said, Focus members were still a long way from the top of the decision-making tree, since ratification for agreed decisions still had to be controlled at a level above that of the MHAG, a process to which Focus did not have access.

In a more positive light, social exclusion had been reduced for members in the following ways.

Reducing social exclusion

- **Building confidence:** Users felt that mental illness had knocked their confidence. Having a voice at a senior level, and seeing unpopular decisions reversed had made them feel valued citizens and had given back a semblance of autonomy and control. This is a key aspect of increasing social inclusion.
- **Decreasing isolation:** Service users felt that they had become isolated by their illness. The social events and networking with other users and allies reduced isolation and also widened social networks, which have been shown to be significantly smaller amongst mental health service users (Buchanon, 1995).
- **Educating the public and reducing 'otherness':** Focus members felt that by being seen to be active campaigners they challenged stereotypes about what people with mental health problems could and could not do. The group felt that by working alongside the MHAG, they would become more active, more challenging, and less compliant in the coming year.

Conclusion

Multi-agency planning is necessarily complex and bureaucratic. It is difficult to persuade people that their participation will result in real changes. It seems particularly hard to agree priorities with the key players and obtain funds to develop new mental health or substance misuse services. For instance, regeneration agencies do not automatically have access to health and social care forums and vice versa.

Moreover, there are structural barriers that can prevent service users and staff having an equal voice in this process. It is perhaps a sad reflection of users' experiences in Hastings and Rother that they felt like a lone voice within the MHAG and more powerful outside of this forum. Despite this, the consensus which has occurred through the primary care trust involvement in a defined geographic locality, coupled with a commitment to mental health and substance misuse has resulted in the improved delivery of local services, better multi-agency working and significant service developments.

 © THE SAINSBURY CENTRE FOR MENTAL HEALTH, 2002

Key points

In Hastings

- Primary and secondary mental health services meet together on a regular basis with service users to review and plan provision.
- Service users are kept informed via a range of methods and have a similar range of ways to contribute their views.
- The authors spent time with a group of users to find out their views on the strengths and weaknesses of the current system for user participation.
- Planning for mental health is linked with regeneration, community safety, and education strategies.

© THE SAINSBURY CENTRE FOR MENTAL HEALTH, 2002

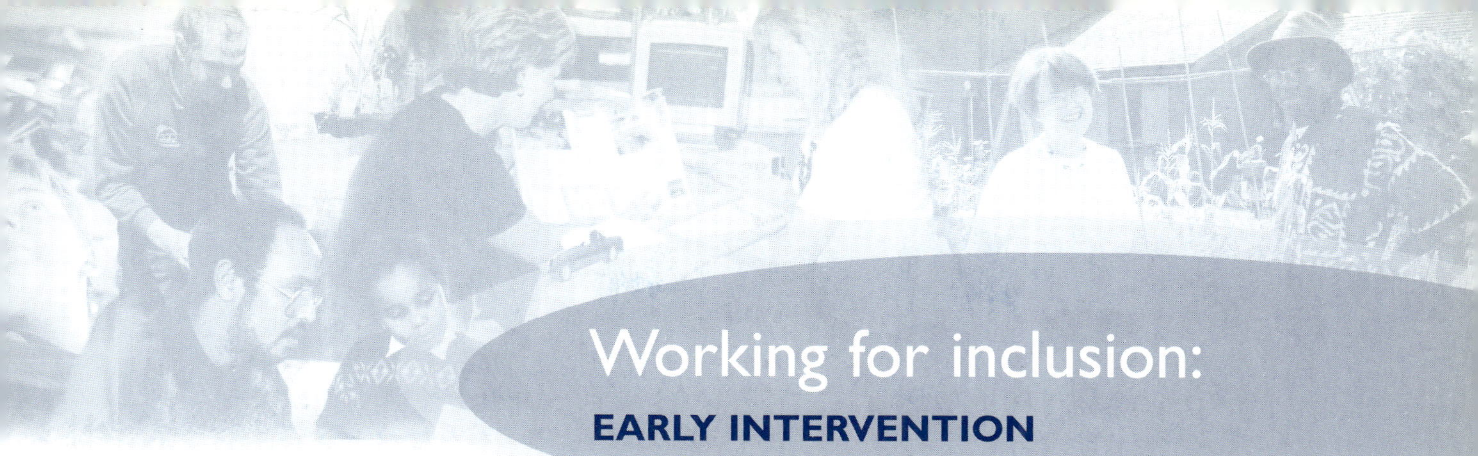

Working for inclusion:
EARLY INTERVENTION

Ruth Marriott

Background

In 1999 Plymouth NHS Trust in conjunction with Janssen-Cilag (a pharmaceutical company) conducted a local audit and found that there was an under-representation of young people aged between 16–25 identified with psychosis. It has been argued that early treatment and support will *"minimise later relapse, social disability and adverse psychological sequelae"* (Department of Health, 1998b).

Evidence from North Birmingham and the Early Psychosis Prevention and Intervention Centre, Australia suggests that early intervention services lead to better engagement in treatment. In contrast: *"The evidence shows clearly that treatment reluctance is substantially increased if first contact with services involves putting you in hospital against your will, giving you treatment you don't want, having major drug side effects and being in an intimidating setting."* (Linszen and Birchwood, 2000)

In Plymouth, discussions between statutory and voluntary sector services had identified the need to fill this gap to meet young adults' needs and ease the often difficult transition between mental health services for children and adults. Two key issues were appropriateness and accessibility of service provision for young people.

The existing Youth Enquiry Service (YES) was identified as the most appropriate setting where an early intervention service could be integrated into a holistic youth service, reducing the stigma attached to seeking help. Health Action Zone Innovations funding was obtained to establish a project called Insight within YES and it is hoped this will become a permanent project. Staff from the Sainsbury Centre for Mental Health are conducting a two-year external evaluation of the service.

The Youth Enquiry Service (YES)

YES has ten years' experience of working with young people on a range of issues. Its holistic, individual approach offers young people between the ages of 13 and 25 access to a range of youth friendly services.

 © THE SAINSBURY CENTRE FOR MENTAL HEALTH, 2002

Based in the city centre with street level access, young people can walk into the service without needing to identify themselves as seeking psychiatric help - they could be approaching any one of the services available. Its confidential, non-judgemental approach enables young people to build relationships with workers on their own terms. All services are offered on a voluntary basis and there is no compulsion for young people to use this service. Services on offer include:

- the Junction – a sexual health clinic and drop-in;
- counselling;
- accommodation and benefits advice;
- mentoring;
- child and youth advocacy;
- personal development programmes;
- Sure Start plus, working with teenage parents and pregnant teenagers;
- Insight – the early intervention psychosis service.

In addition to staffing the shopfront premises, the Insight team undertakes outreach work in Plymouth's communities and schools.

It was important to ensure that in its development Insight was viewed as a YES service that was fully integrated into the mainstream activities of the organisation. It was also important to ensure that other agencies in the city viewed the service in this way and did not see it as an outreach service of statutory adult mental health services.

One commentator has asserted that traditional settings *"are usually aversive and shabby, drug therapies are used crudely, and an individual approach is rare"*. He argues: *"For young people to use health and community services, they must not only be accessible but 'youth friendly'. This can be done by co-locating them with other youth activities and venues where fun and leisure activities are taking place."* (McGorry, 2000)

The Insight team and the service

In trying to minimise the barriers young people face when they have complex needs, we work as a team and collaborate with health staff seconded to work with Insight and other professionals in touch with the young person. The core team consists of a health services manager (up to half time, depending on the development work needed); four key workers (two with YES and two seconded from the NHS Trust); a consultant psychiatrist (one day a week); community psychologist (half a day a week); group worker (half time) and administrator (half time).

 © THE SAINSBURY CENTRE FOR MENTAL HEALTH, 2002

Insight works with young people aged 16–25 with first episode psychosis. The key principles established were that the service would:

- cross agency boundaries and develop integrated ways of working that would limit agency barriers;
- be delivered via a street level youth agency enabling young people to access the service directly and so be provided in a non-stigmatising environment;
- offer a variety of interventions including health, social and psychological support;
- maintain contact with young people for approximately two years – if young people need further mental health support, the project will link young people into adult mental health provision and enable them to make this transition effectively;
- never close – the service is accessible seven days a week, 24 hours a day;
- through a combination of work at the base and in the community, aim to ensure equality of access across the catchment area.

Referral

Insight has been active since July 2000. In the first nine months we received 51 referrals; 19 of these have been self-referrals, the rest have been referred from health services, social services, education or the voluntary sector.

People who are eligible for the service must have been diagnosed with first episode psychosis within the last twelve months, or there must be signs that such a diagnosis might be made. Young people are initially assessed and build relationships with team workers over a month. At the end of this period, we discuss with the young person the best way forward, either with Insight, YES projects or other mental health provision in the city.

The approach

Central to the approach used within this service is the need to:

- engage with young people on their terms;
- enable them to make sense of their mental distress within their life experience, including family, relationships, culture, and the wider community;
- develop coping strategies, de-stigmatise mental illness, ensure that young people can increase their quality of life and remain integrated and active participants within their sense of what community means to them.

 © THE SAINSBURY CENTRE FOR MENTAL HEALTH, 2002

We use a psycho-social approach which includes enabling young people to make sense of their mental distress for themselves, looking at relapse triggers and coping strategies, low level anti-psychotic medication, support to family members, carers or partner and group work.

Our aims are to improve young people's quality of life, prevent admission and readmission to hospital, and prevent young people developing career pathways in the adult mental health system. We work with the young person via the care programme approach to identify holistic responses and personal support.

This includes ensuring that young people are well integrated within their communities and are supported in maintaining active citizenship roles. Siting the service base within a youth agency enables young people to feel less isolated and stigmatised and offers them opportunities to engage in other citizenship roles.

As young people's participation with YES is based on a voluntary relationship the engagement process is extremely important in order to build effective relationships. *"Engagement and rapport building are notoriously difficult problems with people suffering from a psychosis... the acute phase (particularly of first or early episodes) may provide an unrivalled time in which to establish an... alliance."* (Drury, 2000).

Engaging young people who self-refer is by its nature a more difficult process than referrals via another agency that may have some history of contact with the individual (see **box 1**). Self-referrals raise challenging issues for workers and young people to develop active engagement around issues which affect their mental health when they may not recognise that they are having difficulties in this area of their life. For example, a young person may call into YES to find support with accommodation. In addition to the immediate housing issue, the young person may use this contact as a way of testing out the mental health service provided by Insight.

 © THE SAINSBURY CENTRE FOR MENTAL HEALTH, 2002

BOX 1 Engagement

Action: engagement process – building a bridge

- Work on the needs initially identified by the young person.
- Practical resolutions on problems of housing, substance use, relationships or benefits will help to build a trusting relationship that enables you to discuss and address mental health issues.
- This may be the first time a young person has an opportunity to make sense of what is happening to them and their past experiences.
- Ensure that young people are able to make informed choices and give real consent to working with you.
- Think holistically; build in positive integrative opportunities that link them socially with their peers. This might include group events that include opportunities for their friends, rather than arranging events that are exclusive to young people suffering from mental distress.
- Build on current friendship circles – there are often spin-offs in engaging with friends that can enable them to talk about their own distressing experiences that impact on their mental health. This is an opportunity to de-stigmatise mental ill health and enable young people to view mental health issues as a continuum which can affect anyone.

Many young people find it difficult and stigmatising to accept support for mental health difficulties in traditional medical settings. David's story is a good example of the benefits of placing an early intervention service within a holistic youth service.

 © THE SAINSBURY CENTRE FOR MENTAL HEALTH, 2002

Case Study

Colleagues in YES who were becoming increasingly concerned, referred David aged 23, to Insight. When David's mental health deteriorates he finds it difficult to share his distressing thoughts and ideas. To others he may appear bizarre, however, it has become clear that his distress is caused by the constant voices he hears alongside delusional and paranoid thoughts.

Initial links between the Insight team, other workers in YES and David were very informal. It was important not to scare him off by introducing mental health workers to him when he had not voiced these concerns himself.

We had to find a way to engage with him and initially act as a bridge. It took a number of weeks before he felt able to reveal in any detail his thoughts or explain how distressing past events had been for him. This was the first time he had been able to disclose past traumatic experiences.

Engagement process

David had repeatedly contacted YES in the past for two reasons - when his accommodation had broken down and to interact socially with other young people in a safe environment. He had a history of sleeping rough on the streets or in parks, staying in local authority hostels in times of crisis (which led to experiences that negatively impacted on his mental distress) and more recently had been sleeping on a friend's floor. His friend had been taking the vast majority of his DSS entitlement to pay for this, leaving him with very little to live on.

Insight workers began by trying to secure safe and appropriate accommodation for him. This was a difficult and time-consuming process as David found it hard to trust anyone whom he perceived to be in a position of authority. He was caught up in a cycle of mental health issues that disrupted his accommodation and vice versa. Engaging with someone who is homeless is challenging due to the difficulties in not being able to contact them either by letter or phone, and David found it difficult to keep to meeting times. Given his mental health issues the team had to be creative and able to respond quickly. Initially he would often contact the team at crisis point.

Over a number of weeks he began to trust and engage with the team. Workers ensured that David was able to obtain food, receive help with budgeting and obtain support and insight into his psychotic experiences. Our initial approach, which helped him to sort out practical issues, increased his trust of workers and his willingness to engage more fully.

© THE SAINSBURY CENTRE FOR MENTAL HEALTH, 2002

The importance of building trusting, safe relationships – disclosures, delusions and doctors

Over time, David talked about his delusional ideas and the thoughts that occupied most of his waking hours. He began to think about the benefits of seeing the consultant psychiatrist at YES and how anti-psychotic medication might help him. He had fears about possible side effects and concerns about the stigma attached to taking anti-psychotic medication.

Getting to the initial meeting with the psychiatrist was no mean feat. At first, David would initially only see the psychiatrist if he felt he was sufficiently unwell. The team was conscious of treading carefully in order not to scare him off and risk losing contact, as his housing situation and lifestyle were still unstable.

With support and encouragement he finally saw the psychiatrist and the environment and approach used by YES was again crucial in enabling this to happen. Although David continues to find these sessions uncomfortable, he does now feel there is some benefit in them.

A more settled period

David now has a care plan in place and has been supported in applying for a substantial increase in his benefits. This will provide him with additional financial support that will help to improve his quality of life. This was a lengthy process and without YES's support it is unlikely that he would have negotiated the system. Finding appropriate accommodation has also proved to be a lengthy process. However, he has now been offered a permanent place to stay with low-level support and he sees this as an opportunity to put down some roots.

He is aware that this will not be an easy transition for him. We are working with him on his identified goals for the immediate and long-term future as part of the care programme approach. These include enabling him to find appropriate and meaningful employment and increasing his social opportunities.

David has joined group social activities run by Insight - sessions that include a wider social network than just Insight members. Friends are encouraged to join in with the activities and we are in the process of ensuring that this group feeds into the youth forum called 'your shout' run by YES. This enables young people to widen their social networks and have their say in the delivery and development of services at YES, as well as being consulted on wider issues for youth inclusion throughout the city.

 © THE SAINSBURY CENTRE FOR MENTAL HEALTH, 2002

Summary

It is clear from this case study that work with young people on mental health issues is a lengthy process both for the individual and for the community. This is partly due to personal experiences and the need to ensure that young people are not stigmatised, and are able to move forward at their own pace and in meaningful ways. Integration in the life of the community is a key goal for the development of the Insight service, which seeks to break down the barriers that young people face. True inclusion takes time and commitment both from workers and young people experiencing mental distress.

Key points

In Plymouth

- The number of people using mental health services was compared with the local population to identify under-represented groups.
- Services are taken to places already used by young people, including schools.
- The young people's service never closes – it is accessible 24 hours a day, seven days a week.
- Young people can move freely between a wide range of specialists – mental health, housing, benefits, sexual health, parenting, education and training.
- Friends are recognised as important and there are informal opportunities for friends of the service user to participate in activities and get to know the staff.

 © THE SAINSBURY CENTRE FOR MENTAL HEALTH, 2002

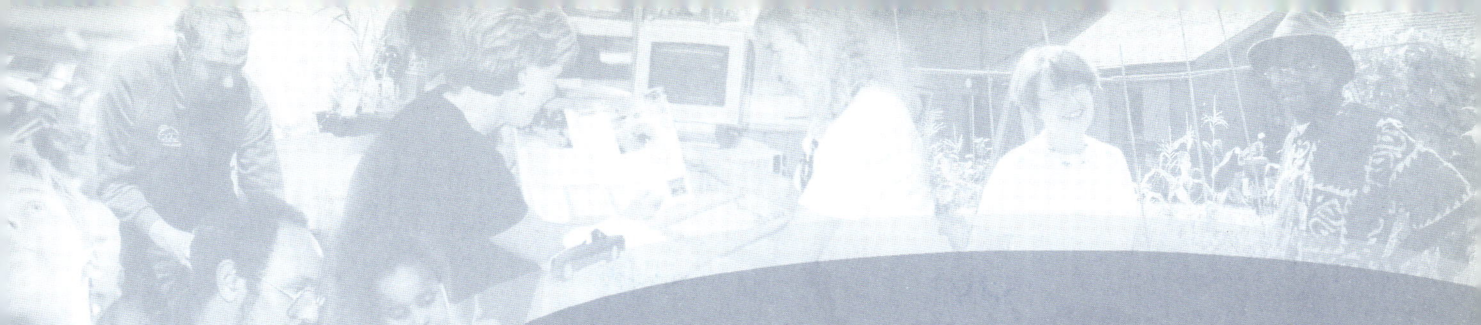

Working for inclusion:
ACUTE CARE

Julie Repper and Rachel Perkins

The idea of 'social inclusion' is often not considered during periods of acute care. Social inclusion is about social roles, networks, relationships and communities whereas acute care often involves time away from communities and networks, social roles and relationships. But, socially inclusive strategies must be prioritised during periods of acute inpatient care to maintain the roles and relationships that are so important for recovery.

> *"During periods of acute distress a person may behave in uncharacteristic, even disturbing ways, they may be unable to meet the expectations of their social, family, work and leisure roles. If they attempt to continue in these roles their relationships may become disrupted and roles jeopardised: friends may avoid them, jobs may be lost, children may be put at risk.*
>
> *"In this situation, a period of admission may help to maintain a person's social roles by relieving them of responsibilities and expectations they are temporarily unable to fulfil. However, in the longer term, admission to a psychiatric ward may lead to erosion of all roles other than that of a mental patient. Lengthy and repeated admissions have been found to lead to smaller social networks, comprising fewer friends and relatives and more professionals and service users." (Holmes-Eber and Riger, 1990).*

This article explores a number of ways in which such socially inclusive activities can become part of the core business of acute services through the development of an inclusive philosophy, an inclusive environment and inclusive practices.

An inclusive philosophy

Developing a 'philosophy of care' can seem an irrelevant diversion on a busy acute ward but it is essential for the whole team to be clear about what they are working towards, how they are working, and what values underpin their work.

All members of the team must have a commitment to helping those admitted resume their former roles, relationships and activities, or develop new ones. Promoting social inclusion is not only important in relation to social functioning, it is also important in maintaining and

 © THE SAINSBURY CENTRE FOR MENTAL HEALTH, 2002

enhancing both physical and mental health. Acute care therefore must look beyond the individual and their symptoms to include their social world and their response to it.

If a team is to genuinely work towards social inclusion of people with serious mental health problems it is important for every member of staff to examine their own attitudes towards people who have mental health problems. Do they really believe in the potential of these people? Would they employ them, live next door to them, welcome them into the family as son/daughter in law? Or do their doubts leak out into their day-to-day work?

These are questions for clinical supervision, but they are also important in establishing a ward team that provides consistency, time, support, warmth and acceptance of (if not always agreement with) the people they are working with.

Numerous first person accounts of the experience of 'madness' illustrate fear of the consequences of mental health problems and psychiatric admission on a person's life. One common response is to 'give up', lose hope and fail to recognise their abilities and potential.

Staff who work on acute wards see people only at the point when their mental health problems are most severe and it is important that their expectations do not become tarnished, so that they fail to recognise skills and abilities and become pessimistic about what a person might achieve. Nothing is more likely to lead to a person giving up than a loss of hope – and it is to this routine under-estimation of potential that 'negative symptoms' such as 'lack of motivation' are increasingly being attributed.

The 'hope-inspiring' competencies of staff are therefore central. It is essential that staff value every person, recognise their potential, nurture their hopes, identify a way towards realising dreams. Thus for example, the desire for a job will help provide the motivation for getting up, washing and dressing on a regular basis, preparing an application, practising for an interview, all of which may fuel the recovery process even if job interviews do not prove immediately successful.

A sense of hope is closely linked with a sense of control of one's difficulties, therefore from very first admission; attention needs to be given to promoting self-management of problems. This involves enabling a person to monitor their own difficulties and crisis/relapse planning to reduce the destructive impact of their problems on their lives.

If a person is able to identify problems early and take the necessary remedial action, then this can decrease the disruptive effect of their problems on their lives and relationships and thus promote their social inclusion. Yet again, this requires staff to trust individuals to make decisions for themselves, to determine the level of help they need, or the dose of medication they feel is most appropriate at that time: to hand over power and see individuals as able and competent rather than passive recipients of care.

© THE SAINSBURY CENTRE FOR MENTAL HEALTH, 2002

If a person is to resume their roles and relationships and rebuild their life, then it is important that acute ward staff attend to the things that are important to service users, even when these differ from what practitioners think is best for them. It is only by ascertaining what people want to achieve and helping them to achieve it that social inclusion can be promoted. Service users have repeatedly been shown to prioritise choice; accessibility; advocacy; equal opportunities; income and employment; self-help and self-organisation (see Read, 1996).

An inclusive environment

While the extent to which the experience of acute admission promotes social inclusion depends largely on the philosophy and practices of the ward team, the physical environment is also important – for staff as well as those who use the service (DoH, 2000). All too often inpatient wards are depressing and demeaning places (Mind, 2001; Standing Nursing and Midwifery Advisory Group, 1999).

Keeping bathrooms and kitchens locked; removing access to cutlery; separate crockery, toilets and sitting rooms for staff; avoiding use of carpets because of the risk of cigarette burns and spillages, all derive from a dehumanising philosophy in which inpatients are neither valued nor trusted.

Psychiatric units often share the features of nearby medical and surgical wards - long corridors, linoleum floors, glass-fronted staff offices from which they can be observed, numerous internal treatment/interview rooms and stifling temperatures. It may not be possible to change the bricks and mortar, but it is not difficult to identify ways in which things can be improved.

Fresh flowers, rugs, bright curtains to provide privacy, artwork, poetry, books in good condition, recent magazines. Areas for women only, areas for smokers, areas where drinks and snacks can be made around the clock as patients wish.

It is vital that the ward environment feels welcoming not only for the individual patient, but also for their relatives and friends. Many people have never been inside a psychiatric facility and retain images of 'madhouses', 'straitjackets' and the like.

If a person's relationships are to be maintained and promoted it is critical that visiting the ward is a pleasant experience and facilities for visitors are inviting and afford some privacy. One room might be designated specifically for this purpose with comfortable chairs, pictures, access to refreshments and information packs about the unit (what it is for, who is who, the routine, answers to common questions etc). There may also be additional details about the nature of mental distress, different types of support/treatment provided and alternative forms of support or therapy that might be helpful.

 © THE SAINSBURY CENTRE FOR MENTAL HEALTH, 2002

But written information is not enough. Seeing someone you love in acute distress is a difficult experience, and family and friends need to feel welcome, with time, information and support from staff when they visit. Suitable arrangements, and support, for children to visit their relatives in hospital must also be considered.

For example, most inpatient areas have a room – a doctor's room, interview room or staff sitting room – that could be transformed into space for visitors. A lot can be achieved with a little creativity and ingenuity.

Inclusive practices

An inclusive philosophy and environment are of little value unless they are matched by socially inclusive practices. In this context inclusion is important in relation to the people who are admitted to the ward, and their relatives, friends, employers, lecturers, and other social contacts.

Involving service users

Socially inclusive practices must start with inclusion of service users at all levels of service provision, from the planning and delivery of individual care, through the operation of the individual ward, and the monitoring and evaluation of services to service planning and development.

Every individual can be involved in decisions about their care through attending the ward round but this can be a terrifying place – particularly for people in acute distress. The presence of someone that the person knows and trusts to accompany them in the ward round may help them to express their wishes and concerns. This may be a friend or relative, but access to independent advocacy may also be important in improving genuine partnership working between service users and mental health workers.

A social inclusion agenda requires that acute wards address the individual in the context of their life: those roles, relationships and activities that are important to the person. This involves extending the remit of assessment and intervention beyond symptomatology. We need to ask people about family members and friends to whom they may be particularly close; whether they have a job; whether there are other people – neighbours, religious leaders, people from the football team in which the person plays or the self-help group of which they are a part – that the person is in contact with. It is only by knowing about the person's social contacts, roles and networks that we can hope to help the person to maintain these over the period of admission.

 © THE SAINSBURY CENTRE FOR MENTAL HEALTH, 2002

Involving family and friends

Although staff on acute settings aim to involve family members, this is often done on an impromptu basis, rarely afforded priority in the urgency of admission, and more frequently done in response to requests from the family.

Staff often have little training or ongoing support in working with families (Fadden, 1997). Certainly families and friends do not feel adequately involved: they do not feel that their accounts are heeded, and their own needs are often unmet.

While plans to keep the family informed of progress and treatment are often intended, these will only be implemented effectively if a clear system of support and involvement of family and friends is planned and agreed by the whole team and implemented throughout the entire admission period. The ward team needs to agree the purpose and value of family involvement, and develop an ongoing assessment and support strategy that is implemented by all staff – including receptionists, domestic staff, the nursing team and psychiatrists.

All need to be positive, supportive and welcoming so that visitors do not feel as though they are in the way. The family may need help to understand the behaviour of the person admitted, how this is managed on the ward, and how they can help.

While a great deal of attention has been paid to the involvement of families in recent years, the maintenance of links with, and support for, friends has been relatively ignored, often leading to the loss of important friendships. On admission, people should be asked about their friendships and offered help to tell their friends that they have been admitted: a person's chances of resuming friendships after admission are jeopardised if they simply 'disappear' from their social networks without explanation. If the person wishes it, friends should be encouraged to visit, staff should be prepared to help the person to explain their problems. It can be difficult for friends to see a person behaving in uncharacteristic and sometimes disturbing ways, and friends need to understand the nature of the person's difficulties if they are to help and support them.

Roles and activities

Given the stigma and discrimination surrounding mental health problems, people often find their discharge from acute care particularly difficult: what do they tell friends, employers, neighbours; how do they explain their absence? An important part of acute care lies in providing support and information to employers, colleges, faith communities and leisure facilities so that opportunities for re-engagement can be enhanced.

 © THE SAINSBURY CENTRE FOR MENTAL HEALTH, 2002

One way of working out how to maintain activities and contacts is to use a weekly diary to record a person's usual routine – before their problems became disabling. This involves spending time with the person discussing the way they spent their week: who they saw when and where, what they did in the evenings, how often they went out, and where to.

This is an important conversation as it confirms that the person is more than just their illness: it goes beyond their problems, and confirms their valued roles and relationships in the community. Many of us do not have buzzing social lives, but we may go to the pub once a week, visit the gym, see siblings once a fortnight, or attend church, the library, weight-watchers. All of these activities count; they give an insight into a person's life outside the ward and are invaluable in planning their support and recovery.

Once significant relationships have been identified, ways of maintaining contact can be planned with the person. There may be a natural wish to hide away from friends and colleagues while in hospital, but continuing contact with the world outside the mental health system is important in reassuring the person that their life has not stopped with admission: that they can still have a life apart from their mental health difficulties, a role other than that of mental patient.

Such continuing contact can be achieved in two ways. First, if given support (some people may want a nurse to be present at first), information and a safe and private place to meet on the ward, friends, colleagues and other social contacts are often pleased to be invited to visit. Second, particularly as the admission progresses, it may be possible for the person to resume some activities from the supportive base of an inpatient setting, rather than try to do this with the relatively lower levels of assistance available after discharge.

Many admissions are repeat admissions, and people may have very few friends and an impoverished routine, with all social contacts associated with mental health services. An admission can be a good time to help people to establish new activities and social contacts or regain those that have been lost. Again it is important to establish their interests, wishes and abilities, to generate ideas and discuss opportunities available in the local area: education, work and training opportunities; social and leisure facilities; support and self-help groups; religious communities and so forth.

Given the importance of work and employment in promoting social inclusion, increasing social networks, enhancing quality of life and promoting mental and physical health, particular attention should be paid to issues of employment or education on acute admission. Employment issues are covered elsewhere in this book so will only be mentioned briefly here. With the person's permission, it may be helpful to: make a specific employment plan; check whether the person has sent a sickness certificate to their employer; liaise with the employer in order to maintain the job; dispel some of the myths associated with admission by contacting their personnel department or occupational health service; or support the person to hand in their notice rather than get sacked.

© THE SAINSBURY CENTRE FOR MENTAL HEALTH, 2002

If the person is not in employment or on a course, or does not wish to return to their former position, then employment or training opportunities should be considered during their admission. For this purpose a detailed vocational assessment should be undertaken (e.g. Becker and Drake, 1993).

It is important to note that such an assessment is not designed to ascertain whether the person is able to work, but to assist in planning the action necessary to enable them to gain and sustain employment and achieve a good match between the job and the person's wishes, skills and problems.

Conclusion

Although current priorities and staffing levels in acute settings often militate against socially inclusive strategies, it is often possible to make some improvements, and to adjust priorities within existing resources. It is quite apparent that the development of inclusive strategies in acute settings could improve services for all involved. Given the evidence that does exist, careful implementation of inclusive practices – in tandem with whole team training, new means of assessment and different use of space on the ward – appears to have the potential to enhance the outcomes of acute care and make work on acute wards more rewarding for staff.

 © THE SAINSBURY CENTRE FOR MENTAL HEALTH, 2002

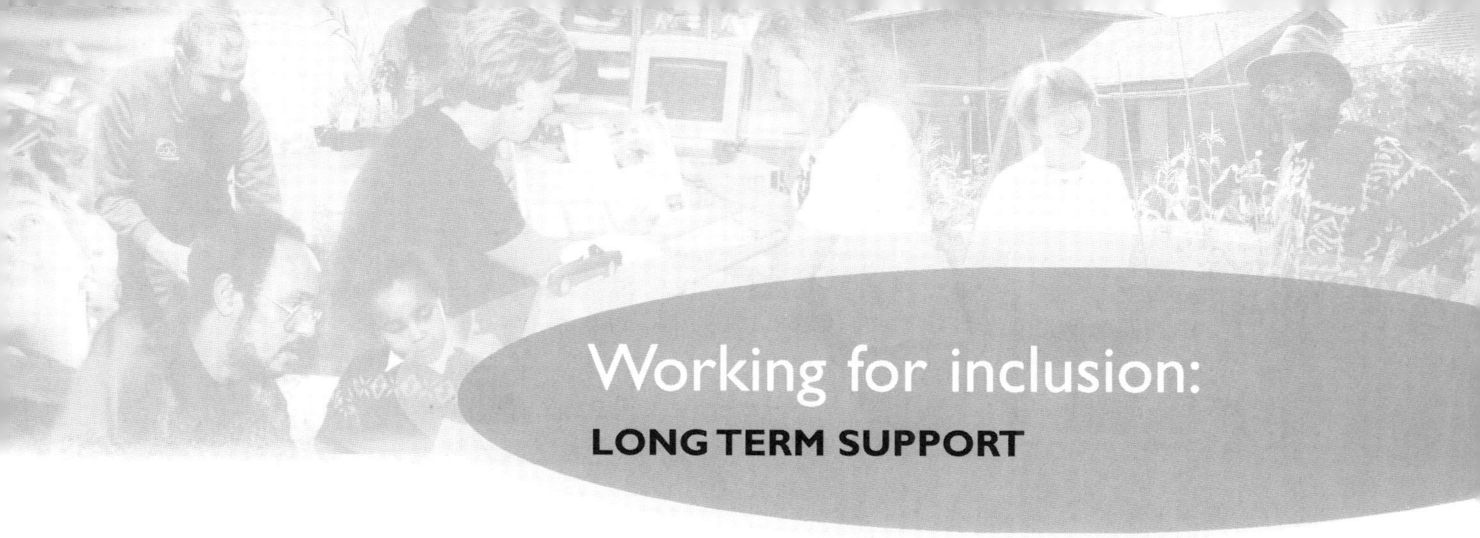

Working for inclusion:
LONG TERM SUPPORT

Andrew Gibb

The *Mainstream* project aims to support users to participate in the wider community and build relationships with people who have no other contact with mental health services. Positive social roles and an improved social life can be expected to enhance the quality of life of participants. *Mainstream* aims to connect users into existing community activities and organisations.

This article is being written at 9.20am in the *Mainstream* office in Liverpool. The walls behind every desk are plastered with posters, postcards and post-its, a reflection of the hundreds of community connections that we have made in the last eight months. Connections with service users, service providers and city facilities in general. Three of the nine full time team members are in the office, which is fine, as only two phones are ringing.

There is a natural resistance to thinking about the past while sitting in a space so full of present requests and concerns. Moreover, the theoretical and philosophical base of the project has now been transformed into real practices with real people, and there is a natural desire to keep this article about real people and real changes. That's not to say the theory behind the project has become redundant. The theory re-aligns us when we have difficult questions about real problems. It underpins the project. So this story of *Mainstream* will start in the present and work its way back to January 2001.

A day in the life: *Mainstream* 8 August 2001

Today, like most days, the bridge-builders (we who help bridge the gap between service users and the mainstream community) are in and out of the office between appointments. Constant communication and networking form the heart of the bridge-builder role. If not out and about, we are engaged in office-bound information gathering, the phone and internet our constant companions.

Today, a community outreach worker called by unexpectedly with a client. He was invited into the office and offered a drink. Paul wants to learn about DJ-ing and doesn't know where to start. The outreach worker had thought of us. Paul doesn't want to be part

 © THE SAINSBURY CENTRE FOR MENTAL HEALTH, 2002

of a big class, though. Something small, informal and basic is desired. Chris, our arts and culture bridge-builder has researched this area before and subject to a referral process can help Paul out. Fulfilling as nearly as possible Paul's particular request is the first aim of the job.

Today two staff have gone out to a local employment service to survey possibilities for several job-seeking service users. Employment service staff were reluctant to hand over information for individuals not present, until the bridge-builders offered their own names as job seekers. Information gathered will be relayed back to service users at personal meetings, along with advice on benefits in relation to work.

Today a staff member visited a mental health furniture project where service users volunteer, gain experience and obtain qualifications. Although referring people to a 'congregated' project like this does not fully reflect the philosophy behind *Mainstream*, we now accept the use of 'stepping stones' as a means to fuller community involvement.

Today a service user attends an oil painting class in the day with support from a bridge-builder. We are about to train our first volunteers who will help people access the activities of their choice, freeing up staff to do more roving work.

In between networking and information gathering, client files must be maintained, letters written, and lunch eaten.

Facts and figures about *Mainstream* August 2001

- 130 people have accessed *Mainstream* for initial advice and information since the project opened.
- There have been 301 follow up contacts with the above group.
- One third of the people referred (31%) have been women.
- Half of referrals (50%) have been on the enhanced care programme approach, a third on standard CPA and the rest were unspecified.

Getting to know you: the referral process

The referral process means getting to know someone and what they want in their life at this time. This involves the following steps:

- *Mainstream* receives a referral form, usually from a mental health service, that has been completed by the client and a keyworker. Our demand for a joint application means that we receive few forms containing prescriptive advice ('I know what will be good for you') from the keyworker. The initial meeting can take place anywhere for the convenience of the client, from their home to a coffee shop.

 © THE SAINSBURY CENTRE FOR MENTAL HEALTH, 2002

- At this meeting the staff member will try to gain as much specific information as possible about the needs of the individual vis-à-vis the activity they wish to pursue. These questions are often of a practical nature (see **box 1**).

BOX 1 Some questions to assess client needs

- What days are you available? Do you prefer a class in the morning or the afternoon?
- Do you want a big or small class, full or part time study, at a college or local community base?
- Is the course for pleasure or to obtain qualifications?
- How will you get there? Do you require personal support to attend the class in the short or long term?
- Are you able to meet any expenses for tuition or materials?
- What do you want the teacher to know about you? Are there any side effects of medication that may affect your performance?

This list is not exhaustive and would obviously change according to the person and the activity specified. It is indicative of our person-centred approach that we try to meet the needs of the individual as nearly as possible. This tailoring means that the client feels more in control of their activity and the potential for continued interest and satisfaction in the activity is maximised. Of course, there is no guarantee that the activity will be pursued or continued, however we will stick with the person until they find what they are looking for.

Monitoring information is recorded. This information is used by the worker as the basis for information gathering on a shortlist of activities and locations that would best suit the client. After eight months the bridge-builders are now familiar with a range of places found to be people-friendly and inclusive. For new locations, staff try to assess them personally with a client in mind. This information will be relayed to the service user via a personal meeting, letter or telephone call, depending on the action needed to initiate the activity.

The bridge-builder may accompany the client on initial or subsequent visits to the activity or meet up to discuss progress.

 © THE SAINSBURY CENTRE FOR MENTAL HEALTH, 2002

Risky business: the place of risk assessment in *Mainstream*

Risk management has been an area of training and debate from the earliest days of our project. However, our attitude to it has changed over eight months. Balancing choice, opportunity and risk is something that all mental health workers have to toil with. It is true to say that in the initial bloom of our project the emphasis was placed more on choice and opportunity than risk. This was a natural stance for a new project to take which required very high levels of open enthusiasm and optimism to create all of its procedures and convert the community and services to its cause.

We are still full of enthusiasm and optimism in August 2001. However, we are paying more attention to risk than we did at the start. This is not due to any calamitous happening. As the project has proceeded we have gained more insights into potential safety issues for our clients, *Mainstream* staff and the community.

We have discovered that we sometimes get conflicting views on the risks associated with a certain client, depending on which staff we talk to. On one occasion we were informed that a client could spend as much time as he wanted in activities with our project and presented no risk to anyone. After several periods of activity another member of staff informed us that the client could be dangerous when unwell and that worker was incredulous that we had not been provided with a more conservative risk assessment. For this type of scenario we have reviewed our risk procedures and have drawn up a *Mainstream* Risk Policy (see **box 2**) outlining responsibilities we all share to promote safety.

BOX 2 Risk policy

***Mainstream* risk policy**

We need a risk policy to enable the client, *Mainstream* and the community to remain safe.

What we expect of you:

- written, clear, precise and up-to-date information associated with the client;
- a written list of signs that might indicate relapse for each individual;
- as medical professionals it is your responsibility to continually assess the person's mental health in relation to their chosen activity and inform us accordingly of the changes.

Continued opposite…

 © THE SAINSBURY CENTRE FOR MENTAL HEALTH, 2002

BOX 2 Risk policy/continued...

What you can expect of us:

- *Mainstream* can offer an information-only service or a more supported service depending on individual circumstances.
- We reserve the right to postpone our services if we believe there is a possible risk to either the client, the community or *Mainstream* staff.
- You can expect us to give you relevant feedback about the person.

The brevity and clarity of this policy is meant to walk the fine line between safety/risk and opportunity. It also places the onus of risk assessment on those who know the individual best. There is no need to introduce the policy in the vast majority of situations where safety risks are not an issue. In the majority of referrals we are usually satisfied with a brief talk about risk with the client and their keyworker.

The origins of *Mainstream*

Mainstream in Liverpool came about as a response to an inter-agency review of mental health services, which revealed the extent of the unmet needs of service users with severe and enduring mental health issues. Fifteen hundred people aged 16-64 with severe and enduring mental health problems in the city were surveyed and results showed that:

- 37% had an unmet need for a meaningful day;
- 26% had an unmet need for friends and relationships;
- 3% were accessing education services;
- 3% were accessing employment services.

In response to these discouraging statistics the Liverpool Health Authority designed a project to address these needs and *Mainstream* was born. 'Imagine', a voluntary sector mental health charity based in Liverpool, won the contract to set up *Mainstream*. Initially the team was to comprise six bridge-builders and a manager.

 © THE SAINSBURY CENTRE FOR MENTAL HEALTH, 2002

Each bridge-builder was to be responsible for a distinct area of life activity:

- arts and culture
- education and training
- employment
- faith and cultural communities
- sports and leisure
- volunteering.

Each team member had a strong background in the area they were chosen for, and were required to help organisations in their field to be more welcoming of people with mental health problems. This is based on the belief that users have a right to access what is available to the whole community, and that these community locations could provide users with a circle of friends and associates unconnected with mental health services.

Early work

During initial training sessions with the National Development Team, staff were sent out to discover inclusive and people-friendly community locations, and analyse why they were good, or not so good. As the team discovered good community locations and allies, we have been creating a database that can be used for future service users. Most of our discoveries come via the particular requests of clients.

In addition to the discovery of good inclusion locations it is also one of the aims of *Mainstream* to provide mental health awareness training where required. June saw our launch conference titled 'Talent going Spare!' which showcased the talent of service users to community representatives.

Aside from discovering community facilities, the early period of the project saw the team descend en masse on all the main mental health services in search of allies and referrals. We were almost universally welcomed for our enthusiasm and common sense in the effort to help people live the lives they wanted. Some seasoned practitioners asked questions we couldn't answer, and pointed to our undoubted lack of experience. We hope that our work demonstrates some real improvements made in some real lives.

© THE SAINSBURY CENTRE FOR MENTAL HEALTH, 2002

Real lives

- J is a fully trained chef who due to severe mental health challenges had been out of activity for two years. With the help of *Mainstream* he now works three shifts per week in one of Liverpool's top restaurants.
- K wanted to do a basic computer course in her local area. After six months of a basic introduction to computers she has signed up for an information technology course and aims to do a counselling course in September.
- P has spent ten years attending his local day centre. As a committed Catholic he has always wanted to attend a Franciscan Lay Order. He has started to attend a meeting of the order in the Cathedral.
- J has just been discharged from a day hospital and wanted to swim as a means of relaxation. She now swims twice a week in the University pool, which is a people friendly location.
- F plays the keyboards. With the help of a bridge-builder he has joined a local band and is playing live gigs.
- G wanted to be involved in physical labour out of doors on a voluntary basis. He now works one day a week with the British Trust of Conservation Volunteers.

Back to where we are: August 2001

The team is still in its infancy. An adjacent health authority wants to replicate the *Mainstream* concept and has funded two additional workers for our team.

New team members force us to reconsider our procedures and habits. In one respect our rapid development all seems a bit fast, but we work as a team and share the load at the busy times. And we can see the fruits of our efforts in the lives of some of our clients. People have set personal goals and with a little information and support some have reached their ambitions. We are far from the finished article as a service, though there are promising signs.

 © THE SAINSBURY CENTRE FOR MENTAL HEALTH, 2002

Key points

At *Mainstream*:

- Each staff member has a specific responsibility to build links with a particular area of community life and has built a thorough knowledge of available people and places.
- Mental health awareness training has been delivered to a variety of community audiences.
- Assessment focuses upon the person's goals, rather than their diagnosis or problems.
- Staff work full time on supporting service users to access ordinary community facilities alongside other citizens.
- Issues of risk and safety for everyone have been reviewed in the context of increasing participation in community activities alongside other citizens.

© THE SAINSBURY CENTRE FOR MENTAL HEALTH, 2002

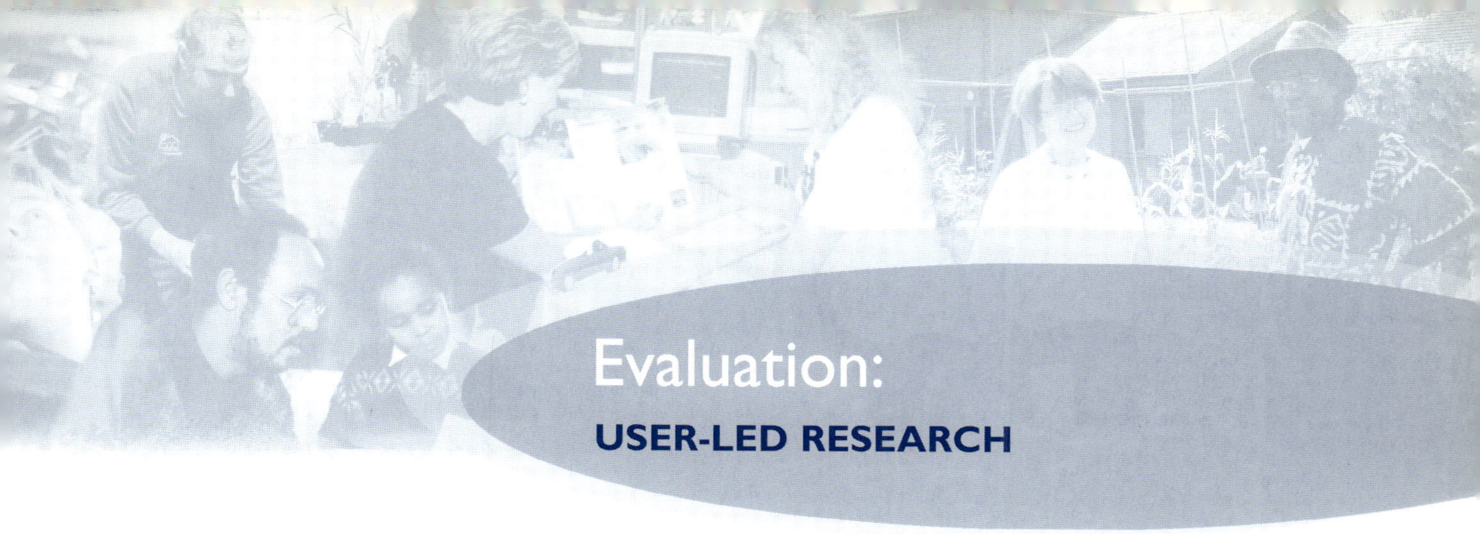

Evaluation:
USER-LED RESEARCH

Alison Faulkner

> *"We are all the primary experts on our own mental health, and about what works for us. We are more than the sum of our individual problems and of the services that we use."* (Faulkner, 1997).

This article is taken largely from the Mental Health Foundation report *Strategies for Living: a report of user-led research into people's strategies for living with mental distress* (Faulkner and Layzell, 2000). It demonstrates the value of listening to mental health service users and survivors about the issues that matter to them in their lives, as well as the value (and a possible method) of including people within the research or evaluation process.

The work of the Strategies for Living project is based on our belief that, as people with experience of mental health problems (or mental distress), we have our own expertise. An expertise frequently overlooked by those involved in the planning and provision of mental health services. We also believe that we are more than the services and the treatments that we use or receive – that we have a myriad of different strategies or ways of managing or dealing with our distress. The research reported here was one element of the three-year project, which also supported other service users and survivors to carry out their own research – and continues to do so.

The primary aim of the research was to build on the evidence from the survey *Knowing our own Minds* (Faulkner, 1997) and to develop a more comprehensive and in-depth body of knowledge about people's strategies for living with mental distress. *Knowing our own Minds* could really only scratch the surface of this knowledge and expertise. Face to face interviews with people would enable us to understand in more depth the reasons and meanings behind different supports, sources of help, treatments and strategies. The aims of the research were to:

- explore people's experiences of different treatments and therapies in order to find out what people find helpful and why, and to explore common themes emerging across the different approaches adopted;
- focus throughout on identifying and understanding people's personal and self-help coping strategies.

 © THE SAINSBURY CENTRE FOR MENTAL HEALTH, 2002

The research process

A key principle throughout the project has been to ensure that the work is grounded in the issues considered important by mental health service users and survivors, and carried out by service users/survivors. The process of doing the research has been considered to be as important as the results, and this has meant that everyone involved has striven to uphold principles of empowerment, consultation, involvement, equal opportunities, respect and confidentiality.

The research process itself was designed to ensure, through both process and content, that users of mental health services are fully involved in determining the direction and implementation of the research. We also aimed to disseminate messages widely and to keep participants informed of the progress of the research. We documented the progress of the study in order to ensure that the work continues to reflect the priorities of service users and is true to its goal of empowerment through involvement and consultation. Thus, we did the following:

- engaged an active advisory committee of mental health service users and survivors from most of the major groups and networks to help us in decision-making and networking activities;
- recruited interviewers and researchers who had experience of mental distress and/or of using mental health services;
- initiated a UK-wide consultation process to ensure that our work was grounded in the current concerns of mental health service users and survivors;
- took an open and reflexive approach to the research.

In the book, *Doing Disability Research*, Barnes and Mercer (1997) say that emancipatory research in the disability context should be enabling rather than disabling, and that it should be 'reflexive' and self-critical. For the research to be 'reflexive' we need to honestly examine the ways in which our identity as researchers affects the research we do and the interpretations we make of that research.

We aimed to do this by reflecting upon the research and how we undertook it. One of the ways we did this was to tape a discussion between us all as interviewers, in which we each reflected on the experience and how we felt about it. We also invited individual contributions for the report from those who took part in the project, giving our own perspectives on the interviewing process, the people we interviewed and some of the painful and thought-provoking issues they raised.

Interviewing is not a neutral undertaking. It is an activity that usually takes place between two individuals, one of whom is the interviewer and the other the interviewee; one will ask the questions and the other will provide answers insofar as they are willing to do so. This sets up a situation where the two people are unequal for the purposes of the interviewing activity, but they may be unequal in other ways too.

Perhaps the interviewer is paid to do the job, middle class, male and white, and perhaps the interviewee is female, unpaid, Asian and working class. There are many other possible differences and similarities between the two people, but there should always be an awareness of the power relationship established from the start of an interview.

One way of potentially reducing the strength of the power relationship between the 'researcher' and the 'researched' is for key aspects of their identity to be shared. In this project, all of the researchers, interviewers and interviewees shared one thing in common: their experience of mental distress and use of mental health services. Our research is as much about our own experiences as it is about the experiences of others (see Vernon, 1997; Beresford and Wallcraft, 1997) in that we too are living with, or have lived with, mental distress. In this respect, disability research is following trends in social research where it has become commonplace to match interviewers to the interviewee's culture, ethnicity and/or gender. This does not remove the power differential between two people where one is the interviewer and the other the interviewee, but it challenges the conventional 'objective' approach to research. It accepts that our identities, as interviewers, can have an effect on the interviewing process.

The way in which the research project arose out of the current concerns of mental health service users and survivors, but also within an established user-led framework at the Mental Health Foundation, reflects our concern to challenge the social relations of research production (i.e. between the researchers and the researched) and crucially, concerning who benefits from the research.

In addition, as users of mental health services, we and our interviewees may have had many difficult experiences of being 'interviewed' in the interests of mental health services, which adds another potential layer of difficulty to the interview. In this project we wanted to know if we would be able to ameliorate this in any way, and enable people to open up about their experiences and views. We identified ourselves as users/survivors of mental health services in the information sent to the people we interviewed, and reiterated it as we introduced ourselves in person.

 © THE SAINSBURY CENTRE FOR MENTAL HEALTH, 2002

We also aimed to reassure people that we were not simply gathering information from them, but were engaging them in a process of discovery and, hopefully, of constructive dissemination. We took additional information about the project to the interview, as well as a list of potential sources of help and advice, and we offered people the opportunity to be on our mailing list to receive our newsletter and information about the progress of the research.

We also emphasised that the information would be used to influence mental health services and professionals, and act as a resource for people with similar difficulties. The aim is to undertake 'research where it will be of some practical benefit to the self-empowerment of disabled people and/or the removal of disabling barriers' (Priestley, 1997).

The research findings

In one of the early discussions with the interviewers, it was suggested that a key finding of the study might be that 'everyone is different'. It is certainly true that the complexity of things that people find helpful in their lives, and the reasons they do so, suggests infinite variety rather than any easy categorisation. However, some strong themes emerged across these differences that enable us to learn some general principles about living and coping with mental distress.

People talked about what they found 'most helpful' in slightly different ways, depending on where they were in relation to their illness or distress at the time of the interview. A number of people described the way in which the value placed on any form of support might vary over time. Different things could be helpful at different times, depending on the nature of change within the illness or distress, and also on the experience gained by the person.

The following broad categories help to describe these different roles, but also demonstrate the immense variation within those roles that could take place between individuals.

On-going survival strategies might include the value and significance of financial security, a sense of belonging and acceptance found in the company of like-minded people, work or daytime activities, physical exercise or the support of a religious faith. Taking control through personal and self-help strategies is another survival strategy, as is enjoyment found in a variety of different interests and activities.

Crisis or life-saving strategies might include contact with friends or professionals, medication and mental health services, the presence of children as a reason for living, the ethos of a religious faith, or an activity such as artistic expression or sport that can capture the attention away from self-destructive or negative thinking.

 © THE SAINSBURY CENTRE FOR MENTAL HEALTH, 2002

Symptom management might be achieved through the appropriate use of medication, through alternative strategies to control voice hearing, such as sport and physical exercise or listening to the radio or Walkman, and through strategies developed through talking therapies.

Healing strategies might be found through healing and complementary therapies, religious and spiritual beliefs, and through the development of personal strategies to achieve peace of mind.

The strategies

- relationships with others, including family, friends, other service users/people with similar problems, mental health professionals, counsellors/therapists, people encountered in day centres, drop-ins, and voluntary sector projects;
- personal strategies, including finding peace of mind, thinking positively and taking control;
- medication;
- physical exercise;
- religious and spiritual beliefs;
- money;
- other activities including, hobbies and interests, information, home and creative expression.

People

The overwhelmingly predominant theme running through people's 'most helpful' supports was the role and value of relationships with other people, in all of their different forms. For some people, it was individuals, family or friends, whilst for others it meant the company of people encountered through local day centres or self-help groups. For still others, the important people in their lives were mental health professionals: counsellors or community psychiatric nurses, support workers or social workers.

One important issue that deserves attention is the relative absence of mental health services and treatments from this section. Mental health services and treatments played an important role in the lives of many people. Medication, when prescribed appropriately, could relieve symptoms and improve mood, and there were a number of mental health professionals who received special mention for the support and the services they provided.

 © THE SAINSBURY CENTRE FOR MENTAL HEALTH, 2002

In this study, however, the most important sources of help remained predominantly outside of the statutory mental health services. However, voluntary sector projects, some of them local Mind associations, some of them mental health projects serving African Caribbean or Asian people, and some of them addressing particular life experiences such as sexual abuse, received enormous and grateful praise.

To understand the 'most helpful' issue in more depth, it is important for us to explore the reasons why these particular supports, people or activities were found so helpful or most important to people, and to look for any common themes that occur across the different factors.

Acceptance

It is clear from listening to the people we interviewed that the stigma and discrimination experienced in relation to mental illness made the acceptance of others a vital element of their survival, and frequently a means of achieving self-acceptance. Many people found coming to terms with distress and diagnosis a long and difficult process. The support and acceptance of others provided a lifeline to survival.

The issue of stigma and discrimination has been highlighted elsewhere (Rose, 1996), and most recently in the Mind Inquiry report *Creating Accepting Communities* (Dunn, 1999). The interviews reported here suggest that many people experiencing mental distress seek out and create their own 'accepting communities', whether among friends or family, or among other people with similar experiences or a shared identity. Where they cannot do so, or are prevented from doing so, we can only reflect the isolation and social exclusion that result.

> *"[Drop-in] is like a safe haven really, from out there…they are just accepted for the person that they are, underneath the illness. That really is the key to it all here."*
> (Faulkner and Layzell, 2000)

Acceptance – or inclusion – was very often found in the company of others who shared similar experiences, or who shared a key aspect of an individual's identity. Some people had discovered the value of shared experience through self-help groups addressing a particular aspect of mental distress, such as sexual abuse or depression, whilst others had discovered it through voluntary sector projects, drop-ins or day centres, where they had met 'like-minded' people.

As much as the frequency with which this theme recurred, it was the strength and passion with which it was expressed that caused it to stand out for us. For some people, finding others who had experienced something similar to them was in itself important, because

© THE SAINSBURY CENTRE FOR MENTAL HEALTH, 2002

they had previously felt alone with their experiences, and now were able to find reassurance and affirmation of their experiences in the company of others.

There were additional issues of racial, cultural or sexual identity for some of the interviewees, which it was important for them to share with the people from whom they sought help. This support was most frequently found through culturally specific voluntary sector projects, such as Asian or African Caribbean day centres or projects. It is significant that many of the Asian and African Caribbean people we interviewed had experienced very little, if any, help outside of these projects; as one Asian woman put it: *"Only (this project) has helped me. No one else has ever helped me."*

Strategies for living phase II: the UK network

Alongside the research reported above, the Strategies for Living Research Support Project supported six small research projects undertaken by service users and survivors, providing training and support over a two-year period.

Out of this work came three new publications (Nicholls, 2001; Malpas and Weekes, 2001; Webb, 2001), with a further three to follow. Following this experience, we were successful in obtaining funding for a further three years, to extend the work around the UK, again from the National Lottery Charities Board (now the Community Fund).

The second phase is designed as a UK network of projects, to be supported by a team of three research support workers based in London, Glasgow and Cardiff. At the time of writing, adverts for the new grants and training opportunities are being widely disseminated, with the aim of starting the projects in the autumn of 2001. Research by, with and for mental health service users is growing in both influence and status.

> *"So many people feel that research is done to them…(user-led research) is all part of the rising tide of empowerment really, people feeling more in control of what they do."*
> (Service user researcher, Strategies for Living Research Support Project)

Key points

- How are service users involved in setting the research questions and designing the research process?
- How are you negotiating the power imbalances that often characterise the interviewer/interviewee relationship?
- How will service users benefit from the research? Will anyone else benefit?
- Many of the people interviewed in this study reported that they found the most important sources of help outside the statutory mental health service. How are local mental health services supporting people to utilise these alternative sources of help?
- Culturally specific projects were reported as very valuable. Is this need met in your locality?

 © THE SAINSBURY CENTRE FOR MENTAL HEALTH, 2002

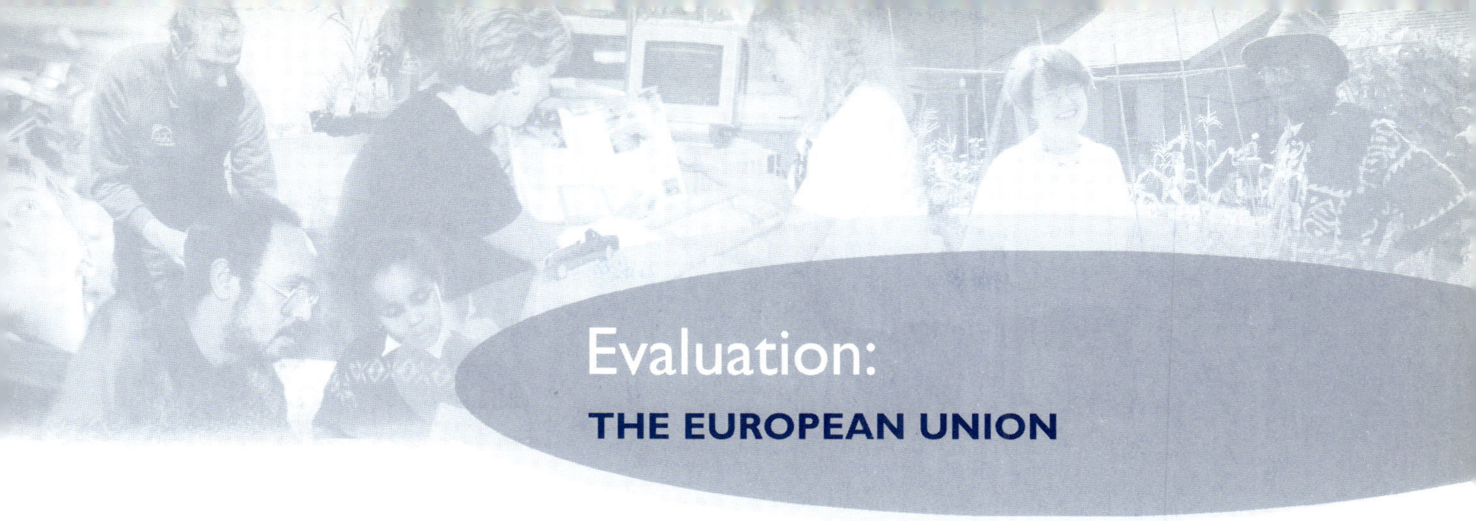

Evaluation:
THE EUROPEAN UNION

Peter Rainford

The European Union (EU) has had a longstanding interest in inclusion issues, usually framed as 'combating social exclusion'. For example in 1989 the European Council adopted a resolution combating social exclusion, which stressed *"That combating social exclusion may be regarded as an important part of the social dimensions of the internal market."*

A variety of definitions of social exclusion and the factors which affect it have appeared in Commission documents over the years.

Amsterdam Treaty May 1999: combating social exclusion

The Amsterdam Treaty included a specific article on the fight against social exclusion and provided the impetus for creating a European Social Inclusion Policy. This article is now enshrined within the *Treaty of the European Union* under article 137. The relevant extracts state:

> *"The Community shall support and complement the activities of the member states in the following fields…*
>
> - *the integration of persons excluded from the labour market;*
> - *equality between men and women with regard to labour market opportunities and treatment at work.*
>
> *"The council…may adopt measures designed to encourage co-operation between member states through initiatives aimed at improving knowledge, developing exchanges of information and best practices, promoting innovative approaches and evaluating experiences in order to combat social exclusion…"*

 © THE SAINSBURY CENTRE FOR MENTAL HEALTH, 2002

Lisbon Summit March 2000: promoting social inclusion

At the Lisbon Summit of the European Council in March 2000 the EU set itself a new strategic goal for the next decade:

> *"To become the most competitive and dynamic knowledge-based economy in the world capable of sustainable economic growth with more and better jobs and greater social cohesion."*

An overall strategy was adopted to achieve this objective. It has three strands, one of which is aimed at:

> *"Modernising the European social model, investing in people and combating social exclusion."*

The Lisbon Summit papers refer for the first time to promoting social inclusion, rather than combating social exclusion. There is a commitment to reduce the numbers of people living below the poverty line and in social exclusion in the union over the next decade and to set targets to achieve this. The current level is described as "unacceptable".

There is recognition that whilst the knowledge-based economy provides tremendous potential for reducing social exclusion it also brings risks of widening the gap between those who have access to the new knowledge and those who are excluded. It goes on to say that the best protection against exclusion is a job.

The key points

Policies for combating social exclusion are to be based on an open method of co-ordination through combining National Action Plans.

The Council and the Commission are to:

- Promote a better understanding of social exclusion through exchanges of information and best practice and on the basis of commonly agreed indicators to be established by the High Level Working Party on Social Protection.
- Promote social inclusion via member states' policies covering employment, education and training, housing and health, and through use of the present EU structural funds.
- Develop priority actions aimed at specific target groups (e.g. minority groups, children, the elderly and the disabled), with member states choosing these actions according to their particular situations, and reporting subsequently on their actions.

 © THE SAINSBURY CENTRE FOR MENTAL HEALTH, 2002

Nice Summit (December 2000): objectives & National Action Plans

The Nice European Council endorsed the work carried out from Lisbon and in particular adopted the idea of National Action Plans on Social Inclusion across the EU. The Action Plans will cover a two-year period and the first draft plans, covering 2001–2003, were to be submitted by member states by June 2001.

The following key goals were adopted at Nice with a view to making a substantial impact on the eradication of poverty and social exclusion by 2010:

- to facilitate participation in employment and access by all to resources, rights, goods and services;
- to prevent the risks of exclusion;
- to help the most vulnerable;
- to mobilise all relevant stakeholders.

It is worth noting that disabled people are specifically mentioned in relation to goals two and three. People with mental health problems are counted as disabled within this framework.

In addition, the Council and the European Parliament are examining a Commission proposal to establish a Programme that will co-ordinate the National Action Plans and promote co-operation between member states. This programme is expected to start from January 2002.

Discussions between the Commission and member states on the National Action Plans have been taking place since July. A joint report is scheduled to be submitted to the European Council at Laeken on 14 December 2001 for adoption.

The UK National Action Plan on social inclusion

Below is a short summary of the policy context and framework of the UK Plan. A full version of the Plan, and indeed all other EU member states National Action Plans on Social Inclusion, can be downloaded from www.europa.eu.int by clicking on employment and social affairs.

 © THE SAINSBURY CENTRE FOR MENTAL HEALTH, 2002

Policy context

The UK Plan states that:

- The National Action Plan reflects the UK's existing strategy against poverty and exclusion, and draws new impetus from the common objectives agreed by the Nice European Council.
- The UK government's commitment to overcoming social exclusion lies at the core of its political programme. However, promoting inclusion is not a matter for central government alone. The success of the UK's inclusion strategy will depend crucially on the contributions of local authorities, the voluntary sector, the social partners and individuals working in their own communities.
- It is important to note that the UK has moved further away from being a unitary state and therefore joint and complementary working between the different tiers of government is key. More detailed information on the nature of devolution in Scotland, Wales and Northern Ireland is set out in Appendices of the UK Plan.

Policy framework

In broad terms the goals pursued by UK policy are:

- preventing social exclusion happening in the first place – by reducing the numbers who go through experiences that put them at risk, or targeting action to compensate for the impact of those experiences;
- re-integrating those who become excluded back into society, by providing clear ways back for those who have, for example, lost their job or their housing or missed out on learning;
- getting the basics right – delivering basic minimum standards to everyone in health, tackling crime, education, employment, in-work income and retirement income.

These goals are pursued by a strategy based on the principles of:

- structuring policy interventions around a life cycle approach, where necessary to meet individual need;
- tackling failing communities and the needs of other excluded groups and people;
- mobilising all relevant actors in a joint multi-agency response;
- tackling discrimination in all its forms, wherever it occurs;
- ensuring all policy formulation is evidence based.

This National Action Plan sets out the UK's plans to apply these principles in pursuit of the common objectives agreed by the Nice European Council.

 © THE SAINSBURY CENTRE FOR MENTAL HEALTH, 2002

Key points

It is likely that the European perspective on social inclusion will become increasingly important over the next decade because:

- The Commission and member states will refine and develop National Action Plans.
- The Commission will develop indicators and outcomes to measure and compare social inclusion across the EU.
- Practitioners will be able to use the European Social Inclusion agenda to influence national and local policy and practice.
- The Community Initiative proposed by the Councils at Lisbon and Nice will provide a new source of funds for actions around social inclusion. Although Community Initiatives represent only five per cent of the EU structural funds they are applicable throughout the European Union and will therefore be available for actions throughout the UK.

 © THE SAINSBURY CENTRE FOR MENTAL HEALTH, 2002

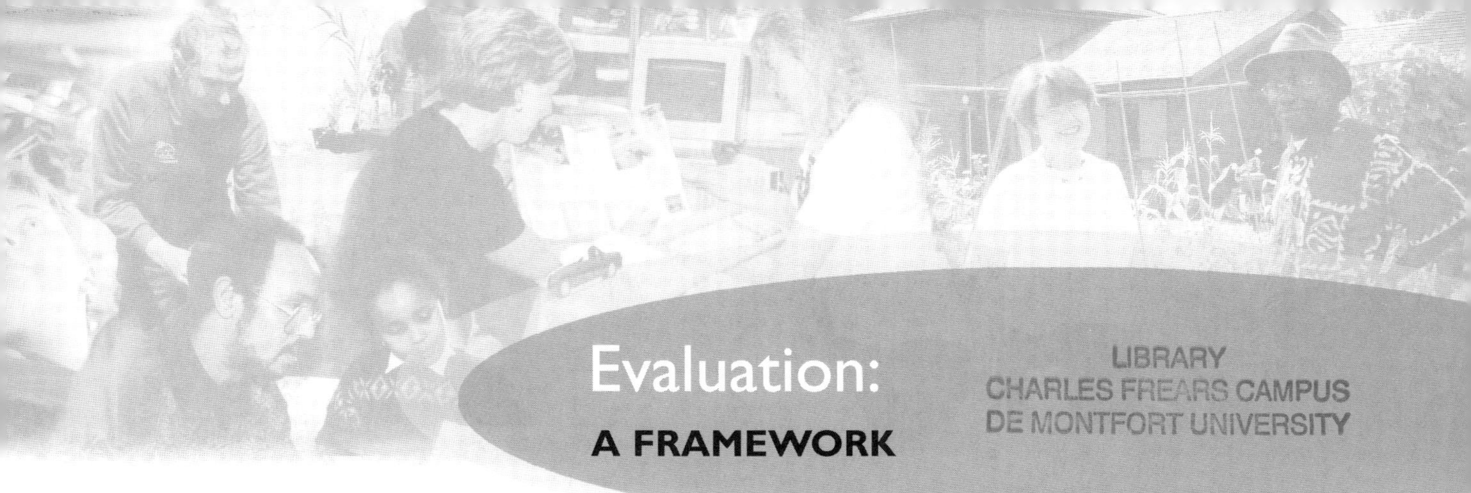

Evaluation:
A FRAMEWORK

LIBRARY
CHARLES FREARS CAMPUS
DE MONTFORT UNIVERSITY

Peter Bates and Julie Repper

Over the past decade, there has been increasing recognition of the disabling effects of social exclusion. Government policy has explicitly linked the work of different agencies (housing, environment, health, social services, the church) in the Social Exclusion Unit set up to combat the ill-effects of 'social exclusion', which it defines as:

> "*What can happen when individuals or areas suffer from a combination of linked problems such as unemployment, poor skills, low incomes, poor housing, high crime environments, bad health and family breakdown".* (Social Exclusion Unit, 1999)

Sayce (2000) provides a more precise definition of social exclusion that draws attention to the interactive relationship between impairment and social role. Although this refers specifically to mental health problems, it can be applied to all those who suffer marginalisation and discrimination as a result of impairment – whether it is emotional, cognitive or physical:

> *"... the inter-locking and mutually compounding problems of impairment, discrimination, diminished social role, lack of economic and social participation and disability. Among the factors at play are lack of status, joblessness, lack of opportunities to establish a family, small or non-existent social networks, compounding race and other discriminations, repeated rejection and consequent restriction of hope and expectation."*

As these relationships have become recognised, many organisations have incorporated goals to combat social exclusion in their core purpose, and there has been a welcome upsurge of interest in strategies that strengthen communities, increase social capital and support individuals to live as valued members of a democratic society.

While goals and strategies are an important part of the change process, evaluation is needed to drive that change forward. To date however, evaluation has failed to realise its potential. Here we have set out a framework that we hope will provoke rigorous thinking about how to evaluate an inclusive effort.

We developed this framework in consultation with members of the Inclusion Research Network, an informal group that shares an interest in increasing opportunities for people who are at profound risk of being excluded.

 © THE SAINSBURY CENTRE FOR MENTAL HEALTH, 2002

Most members work in mental health, learning or physical disability services, but the group is not exclusive to these labels. For the network inclusion in society means full access to mainstream statutory and post-16 education, open employment and leisure opportunities alongside citizens who do not bear these labels. The group concentrates on those people who, along with their allies, need to make a focused effort to achieve inclusion. This effort consists of a two-pronged approach of simultaneously re-shaping the community and providing one-to-one support to the individual.

A search of the literature suggests that progress is confined to isolated pockets. For example, Circles of Friends have been used to support children in mainstream education, rather than diverting them into the local special school (Newton and Wilson, 1999).

When it comes to evaluating this activity, one researcher asked family members about their satisfaction with the project (Whitaker *et al.*, 1998), and another examined the pace of learning of the non-disabled pupils who shared the classroom (Bunch, 1997).

While the same principles might apply to an adult entering open employment (family members could support or sabotage, and co-worker productivity could increase or decrease), we know of no studies that have examined these variables. This led us to develop a framework that attempts to describe all the variables that might be captured in an evaluation.

We hope:

- inclusive projects that are planning an evaluation will use the framework to consider which variables are relevant to their purposes;
- readers who detect missing elements in the framework will contact us so that future versions can be more comprehensive (see ***List of contributors*** p265);
- to develop a version which makes detailed reference to the evaluation instruments that have been utilised in other studies;
- to identify gaps where evaluation tools have yet to be developed.

Ethics and philosophy of evaluation

We start with the fundamental question about what the evaluation is for and who owns the work. Whilst traditional science has promoted randomised controlled trials and outcome-based research, this is beset with problems in the field of inclusion. Existing outcome measures simply do not reflect the complexity of inclusive endeavours – which take place with both the individual and her/his multiple communities.

 © THE SAINSBURY CENTRE FOR MENTAL HEALTH, 2002

The multi-faceted nature of work with any individual to achieve their personal goals requires individually tailored approaches that are difficult to specify for the purpose of comparative experimental research. Besides, in an area that is explicitly about inclusion and empowerment, we inevitably favour emancipatory research – an approach that empowers people. Such collaborative methodologies have the advantage of drawing on the skills and experiences of all those involved, in both the development of strategies and their evaluation.

Inclusive approaches are in their infancy; it is only by working with those providing support, influencing local cultures and those receiving it that they can reach their full potential. Definitions of success vary according to perspective: service users, carers, service providers and commissioners all have different ideas of success and these must be taken into account in planning and undertaking evaluation. Participatory action research is one example of such a co-operative endeavour. Case study research, using different types of data collected by and from different 'stakeholders' is another research approach that is consistent with reflecting the views of all parties (see Robson, 1993). For individualised outcome data, personal goal attainment scaling is a method of assessing the achievement of individualised goals (Ottenbacher and Cusick, 1993).

The Strategies for Living project has recently promoted the employment of mental health service users as research staff, and convened a forum for user-researchers (Faulkner, 2000). An increasing number of projects share the design stage of the evaluation with service users, employ users to undertake the evaluation, glean evidence from service user accounts, and involve users as co-authors and conference presenters in disseminating the findings.

Where do we start?

In the following material we have chosen to begin with the person who needs support to engage in a community opportunity. In doing so there is a possibility that readers will conclude that the entire problem lies with the person who needs support, rather than the environment.

In reality, all the factors that we list are interdependent and none is more or less important than the others. Perhaps we should have begun with an examination of the site of support rather than the focus person. But we had to choose where to cut this wheel and roll out the circumference into a story line with a beginning, middle and an end. So we began with the focus person for the sole reason that this seemed to us to be the simplest place to begin, the clearest way to open up a subject that can become complex.

Despite the considerable research literature on social inclusion, we still know very little about what works. This means that the field is full of untested hypotheses. The clear-headed evaluator will use criteria such as the following to test each assumption that she or he

 © THE SAINSBURY CENTRE FOR MENTAL HEALTH, 2002

makes. However, many of us in the real world are less clear-sighted. We live with working hypotheses and use them to select environments that we anticipate will be successful sites for inclusion.

For example, we guess that a company that respects all its staff will be a good place for a person who needs support to work. As a result of this (untested) hypothesis, we use the criteria to pre-select suitable workplaces and reject others. Practitioners are likely to work in this way, but also deliberately question and test these hypotheses from time to time.

The remainder of this article consists of five major headings that together form our framework for evaluating inclusive projects. Under each heading we have set out a number of questions or issues that could be the subject of formal evaluation.

The focus person

When a person is supported to attend a mainstream school, enter open employment or join the dominoes club at their local pub, we can ask some questions about the person themselves. To obtain a baseline measure of their need for support, we may wish to explore the person's skills, attitudes, self-esteem, communication, social network and relevant history and ambitions. We can ask what support they expect to receive in the mainstream setting, such as the number of hours a jobcoach will work with the person. Support in other settings will be relevant too – the amount of medication or frequency and duration of hospital admissions may reduce when the person moves into a valued role in the community.

As participation in the community-based activity continues, there may be a change in the person's level of skills or difficulties. For example, daytime exercise may improve sleep, reduce the disruptive impact of voice hearing and improve a sense of well-being. Specific landmarks may be passed in the community setting, such as the person obtaining a contract of employment, formally registering as a member of the group, or obtaining a qualification.

New friends and associates may appear in the person's network. The number of attendances, output, earnings or learning gained will give a sense of the person's degree of engagement with the activity. For example, some supported employment schemes log the average hours worked per week, wage rate and tax paid by the focus person.

Finally here, it is worth noting that the adoption of valued community-based roles may not have a uniform beneficial impact. For example, some jobs are so demanding that stress levels increase, diet deteriorates, and friendships are eroded.

 © THE SAINSBURY CENTRE FOR MENTAL HEALTH, 2002

The site

Prior to the start of the community opportunity, support staff will have worked with the focus person to identify suitable activities, locate an appropriate setting and assess its suitability. An assessment of the site will include an initial consideration of the fit between the environment and the person.

In addition to physical and sensory access (ramps, induction loops, adequate lighting and so on) the social and organisational environment needs to be considered. Attitudes, policies, practices, communication networks and appraisal/feedback mechanisms are all important. Do teams have some degree of self-management and are the views of all participants in the setting valued? Is bullying rigorously opposed and are conflicts effectively resolved?

Asking these questions at the site may provide some clues to the focus person about whether s/he wants to participate here. It may also provide indicators of successful placements that inform future inclusive work. Monitoring the site over time may well show that the presence of the focus person has led to changes in policies, practices or attitudes within the organisation.

The new community

This segment examines the characteristics of the group that the focus person is trying to join. Social and demographic indicators may be relevant, as well as some knowledge of the history of the group. For example, a mainstream school that has welcomed children with mobility problems may be less fearful about playground accidents than a school that has not done so.

More importantly, the attitudes, values and knowledge of the particular community will affect the initial experiences of the focus person. Repper and Brooker (1996) found that people with mental health problems experienced a higher level of discrimination in *"established communities, deprived and saturated areas, family centred communities and areas with no previous contact"*. It is important to actually evaluate attitudes, rather than make assumptions. For example, if a person is hoping to join a faith community, then one congregation may connect disability with guilt or evil while another will focus on the precious humanity and gifts of each individual.

Some inclusive projects (such as the Kent scheme described in ***Section Three***) offer training to community audiences, including an assessment of attitudes before and after training. One might also expect that attitudes, values and knowledge will change as the focus person becomes well-known within the setting.

 © THE SAINSBURY CENTRE FOR MENTAL HEALTH, 2002

A deeper exploration of the group might include values and attitudes about disability in general or a particular kind of disability. The extent to which peers know and trust each other, the way in which they respond to newcomers and their sense of affiliation with the setting will all impact upon the inclusive effort. In addition, it may be possible to identify and influence some key opinion-formers who will have a disproportionate impact upon the overall attitude or culture of the setting (Repper and Brooker, 1996).

Finally, some concrete measures of productivity or learning by the co-participants were referred to in the introduction to this article. For example, the reliable attendance of a supported volunteer may spur other volunteers on to keep faith with their commitment to the shared voluntary work.

Family and friends

While there are many good reasons for paying close attention to the focus person and the new setting, other people can have a powerful impact upon the success of the inclusive effort. Some researchers have concentrated upon relatives and the potential for the service user to have a negative impact upon their quality of life (the 'family burden' experienced by the 'carers' in this hypothetical one-way relationship). Whilst we recognise the reality of these findings, we also note that people who need support can be strongly valued by their non-disabled family and friends (Nelson *et al.*, 1992, Newton *et al.*, 1995), and that encouragement from loved ones can make all the difference to the success of a placement.

It would be possible to include a range of indicators that tell us how family and friends are affected by the inclusive effort. Satisfaction and quality of life will be an issue for all family and friends and the general health of some people, especially older family members, may be important. There may be some exchanges of support that are also relevant. For example, the parents may be rising earlier on 'real job' days to provide a wake-up call, but the new job also means that the person can pay for board and lodging.

Brokers

The last group of issues this framework considers is the people who hold power over the inclusive effort. This may include health and social care staff who can make an initial referral; specialist brokers, such as vocational guidance staff or a volunteer bureau adviser; or policy leaders in each setting, such as the occupational health physician. These individuals have the power to initiate a potential opportunity, give reassurance to the person directly managing that inclusive environment, or bring the arrangement to an end.

© THE SAINSBURY CENTRE FOR MENTAL HEALTH, 2002

The wider political context has a strong impact upon brokers. For example, jobcoaching agencies might have experienced a rapid increase in the number of opportunities on offer following the launch of the Disability Rights Commission.

In addition to formal changes in the political landscape, softer changes may also have a serious impact. For example, a minor revision of the funding formula for college courses can have an amplified effect upon the opportunities for people who need learning support. Of course, brokers will have a range of attitudes and values alongside everyone else, so it would be useful to measure their attitudes along with those of other parties.

This article previously appeared in *A Life in the Day* and is reproduced with permission.

Key points

- Does your organisation routinely collect performance management data that includes a measure of the extent to which service users are socially included? What data is collected and who uses it?
- Who selects issues for research? Does the programme include questions about social inclusion?
- Do local services that promote inclusion evaluate their success? Which criteria and methods have been used?
- Develop an action plan for future evaluation. What needs doing and who could do it?
- If you need some help, why not locate people who are interested in conducting research – service users, students within the mental health professions or in other disciplines, or volunteers.

 © THE SAINSBURY CENTRE FOR MENTAL HEALTH, 2002

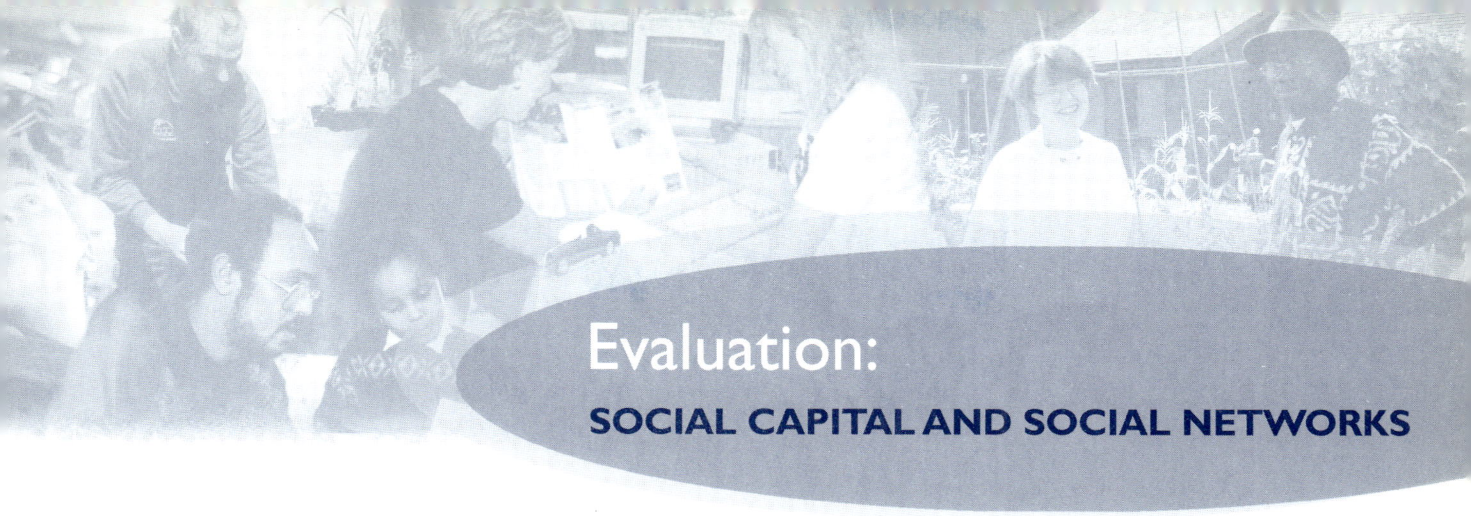

Evaluation:
SOCIAL CAPITAL AND SOCIAL NETWORKS

Sarah Hean

Introduction

Social capital is a valuable concept for mental health services. Providing support often includes helping people participate in networks, while social capital explores the advantage gained by the individual from being part of these networks. Although social inclusion cannot always guarantee that a user will have access to these benefits, social capital and social inclusion are related.

In other words, there is a greater likelihood that socially included individuals have better access to the advantages associated with high levels of social capital. The purpose of the article, therefore, is to discuss the value of social capital as a lens through which health/ social services and community projects that wish to promote social capital may be viewed. The individual user will be the main focus.

The meaning of social capital

Many community-based projects and service providers have the improvement of user social capital as an aim, and plan to evaluate programmes in terms of social capital. It is frequently evident from project reports that social capital is often poorly understood and thought to have a universal meaning, which, as yet, it does not. It is thus added somewhat vaguely into report documents without any clarity of the meaning the reporter has attached to the construct.

To provide an overall feeling of the significance of social capital, a concept analysis of social capital (Cowley *et al.*, 2000) outlined some of the more common understandings of the term, dividing the construct into its general attributes and its component parts as well as the antecedents and consequences. These findings will be summarised in this article, providing examples of questions that can be used in measurement. Hopefully this summary will improve understanding and use of the term in programme design and evaluation.

 © THE SAINSBURY CENTRE FOR MENTAL HEALTH, 2002

Overall definition of social capital

Social capital is an advantage gained through social process.

General attributes

Several general attributes are associated with social capital but five are central. Social capital:

- exists in or through social relationships;
- is dynamic;
- is durable;
- has a function, e.g. it facilitates action; it encourages co-operation and learning or it deepens trust;
- is multi-dimensional.

Social capital is **capital**. Capital is something dynamic that continually changes from one form to the next. It also has a tendency to accumulate and endure. If a project has the aim of improving social capital in post-natally depressed mothers, for example, then describing the project in terms of social support alone implies a static one-off event whereby help is given by one person to another. If, however:

- effective support is provided in a context that fosters trust in the project and its members;
- if this increase in trust encourages the young woman to continue participation in the group, other groups or take up other civic activities;
- the increase in trust has increased the level of involvement of the woman, motivating her into taking on a leadership role;

then one has described a process whereby emotions, attitudes, events and outcomes are linked in a dynamic and sustainable chain. This process describes social capital.

Social capital covers a whole range of situations, ranging from long-term membership of a face-to-face group through to single events such as voting, picking up litter or even taking an interest in local events by reading the local newspaper.

As many aspects of social capital are illustrated vividly through group membership and this is also the area where measurement is most easily tackled, the rest of this article will focus on social capital in the context of a formal face-to-face group.

 © THE SAINSBURY CENTRE FOR MENTAL HEALTH, 2002

However, it is important to remember that a comprehensive assessment of social capital will encompass the broader definitions that reach beyond the confines of one single, isolated group. Each community, group or service under study will exhibit very different levels or forms of social capital and what is optimum in one context, may not work in another.

Each component of social capital will now be discussed with some examples of measurement.

Characteristics of the network

Social capital is created within networks of relationships. The network is, therefore, an important component of social capital and is evaluated in terms of its characteristics. Which characteristics of a network should programme leaders measure and what form should they take to promote social capital?

Network characteristics may be divided into those that relate to the physical characteristics of the network and those related to sentiments or emotions stored within them – the cognitive characteristics (Krishna and Shrader, 1999).

Physical characteristics

Size and longevity of network. Networks may range in size (e.g. a network of two people represented by the relationship between a patient and his/her GP or a huge network such as that formed by the members of Greenpeace).

Networks may vary in duration (e.g. a single visit of ten minutes to a service provider or a Health Action Zone project lasting two years). Measurement of the size and longevity of the network has an influence on the functioning and outcomes of the group as a whole, and thus the social capital accessible to individual members. The optimum size or duration of the project is dependent on the purpose and circumstance of each individual project/service.

Frequency of participation. In general more frequent participation makes it more likely that the individual will benefit from the group. Participation in the network is not confined to physical appearances at network meetings but may also involve other forms of contact (see **box 1**).

 © THE SAINSBURY CENTRE FOR MENTAL HEALTH, 2002

BOX 1 Network contacts

On average, how often, in the last 12 months have you

- Attended meetings of the group?
- Phoned or been phoned by people from the group?
- Emailed or been emailed by people from the group?
- Written to or been written to by people from the group?
- Done some form of preparation for meetings held by the group?
- Done some form of administrative work for the group?
- Met with members from the group outside of group meetings on matters that concern the group?
- Met with members of the group outside of group meetings on other matters (e.g., socially)?

(Adapted from Cowley *et al.*, 2000)

Nature of involvement. Participation alone does not guarantee that the individual will be sufficiently integrated to gain from the network. Assessment of the nature of involvement is, therefore, useful with the assumption that greater levels of involvement are associated with better chances of obtaining the benefits associated with being a network member (see **box 2**).

BOX 2 Where do you fit?

- Are you a leader in the group? Do you consider yourself to be active in the group, such as by attending meetings or volunteering your time in other ways, or are you relatively inactive?

(Adapted from Krishna and Shrader, 1999)

 © THE SAINSBURY CENTRE FOR MENTAL HEALTH, 2002

Number of relationships held in network and ties. The individual group member may know only one member of her network or everyone, and not all relationships may be of a similar strength. A network may have an open structure or cliques may exist of which the individual may or may not be part. Mapping procedures, such as social network analyses, may be of use to understand this context. These features may influence the passage of information between network members and influence who is in the optimum position to benefit from this knowledge (Burt, 1997; Granovetter, 1973).

Hierarchical versus horizontal. Networks may be hierarchical or have a horizontal structure where members are of more similar status and power (see **box 3**). The latter is viewed as favourable in the promotion of trust and co-operation within networks (Putnam, 1993).

BOX 3 Status in group

When there is a decision to be made in the group, how does this usually come about?

- The leader decides and informs the other group members.
- The leader asks group members what they think and then decides.
- The group members hold a discussion and decide together.

(Adapted from Krishna and Shrader, 1999)

To what extent do you participate in this group's decision making?

(Adapted from Narayan, 1998)

Heterogeneous versus homogenous networks. The specific function or benefit gained from a network will dictate whether homogenous or heterogeneous groups are preferable in social capital generation. A heterogeneous group, for example, may make available a more varied source of skills to the network whereas a homogenous group may be bounded together by a common feeling of solidarity based on most members having common characteristics (see **box 4**) (Portes and Sessenbrenner, 1993).

 © THE SAINSBURY CENTRE FOR MENTAL HEALTH, 2002

BOX 4 Others in the group

Thinking about the members of this group, would you say most of them are from the same...

- neighbourhood/village/community
- family or kin group
- ethnic group
- gender
- linguistic group
- religious group etc.

(Adapted from Narayan, 1998)

Formal versus informal networks. Networks may vary from informal, i.e. relationships with friends and family, to the more formal shown by relationships with people at work, with members of a community project or between a client and a service provider (Krishna and Shrader, 1999). Surrounding a formal network are informal networks that are likely to influence its effectiveness.

When measuring social capital, questions for informal networks may need to be very different to those appropriate for the formal setting. Asking, for example, why people chose to join a particular network is an appropriate question to be asked in the formal environment. It is not well received in the informal network setting where reasons for remaining part of a family or friendship network are less well analysed by the user.

Cognitive characteristics of the network. Examples of these features are levels of group cohesion, commitment to and identity with the group and the extent of shared values, attitudes and beliefs (e.g., Krishna and Shrader, 1999). Here is an example (see **box 5**) of some items used in measures of social cohesion.

 © THE SAINSBURY CENTRE FOR MENTAL HEALTH, 2002

BOX 5 Group dynamics

To what extent would you say that...

- People in my group are close knit.
- People in my group do not have much in common with each other.
- You have to take care of yourself first, even at the expense of other people in the group.

(Adapted from Kawachi *et al.*,1999)

Social interaction

Two forms of social interaction may occur within a network being evaluated in terms of social capital: complementary and symmetrical interaction. In complementary interactions, individual A receives help from individual(s) B, B having the capacity and resources to provide this help. In symmetrical interaction, on the other hand, the emphasis is on the collective, with a group of individuals working together towards a common goal (Snijders, 1999). One or the other, or a combination of the two may be suited for different networks of different outcomes. Observation research methods are the most obvious means of measurement.

Trust

Trust is perhaps the most central component of social capital and its measurement has taken various forms ranging from the general (e.g. trust in society and people in general) to the specific (trust in named organisations, government or in other club members). The effect of the group on the development of trust (see **box 6**) which may encourage the user to continue participating, is particularly important when considering social capital. Reapplication of trust questions at staged intervals of the project's lifetime may provide an indication of changes over time.

 © THE SAINSBURY CENTRE FOR MENTAL HEALTH, 2002

BOX 6 Group trust

Generally speaking, do most people in the group...

- act in a trustworthy fashion;
- treat each other unfairly;
- would take advantage of me if they got the chance.

(Adapted from Kawachi *et al.*, 1999)

Resources

Participation in highly cohesive networks where trust between members is high cannot guarantee that positive outcomes associated with membership can be achieved. Appropriate resources within the network and the individual him/herself must be present for this to be achieved.

The external resources of the network can take both physical and more abstract forms, depending on the nature of advantage to be gleaned from social interaction. If the benefit is support in times of financial difficulty, then there must be other members in the group that have sufficient funds to offer this support (see **box 7**).

Alternatively, groups whose goal is emotional or practical support, require other resources more abstract in nature such as provision of information or a variety of counselling skills. External resources also include the willingness of others to assist or co-operate as well as the feelings of common identity and commitment to the group that may facilitate this (Snijders, 1999; Kilpatrick, 2000).

© THE SAINSBURY CENTRE FOR MENTAL HEALTH, 2002

BOX 7 Relations with others in the group

Generally speaking…

- I know people in the group well enough to be prepared to help them.
- If I realised someone needed help in the group I would try and help them.
- I do not feel others in the group are worth helping.

(Adapted from Cowley *et al.*, 2000)

An individual, to be able to seek out support or whatever other benefit she seeks, must have within herself the knowledge of when, whom and where to go for this benefit (see **box 8**), (Kilpatrick, 2000). These have been termed internal resources.

BOX 8 Sources of help

- If you need information to make a life decision, where would you go for this information?
- Sometimes, people have great financial difficulty, because of ill health, a death or loss of a job. Who would you turn to in the group for help?

(Adapted from Narayan, 1998; Bullen and Onyx, 1998)

Norms and rules

The final component of social capital to be discussed is the rules and norms that govern behaviour in the network. Rules tend to govern behaviour in more formal networks and facilitate actions that are conducive to beneficial outcomes for the group as a whole and/or the individual (Collier, 1998). Assessment of how rules and regulations, set down by a service or community project, influence member behaviour and outcomes should be considered.

Norms are less formal than rules and are less well analysed by the people whose actions they direct. Norms of reciprocity, associated with the generation of obligation, are the most common norms discussed by those interested in social capital. One member of a project may help another at some stage in the life of the project and the latter may feel obliged to repay this debt (Coleman, 1988).

Whether this occurs depends on several things, the opportunity to repay the debt being one: a user of a service may never have the opportunity to repay the help of the service provider, for example. Secondly, the strength of the norms of reciprocity may dictate if an obligation is repaid. In the case of service provision, norms of reciprocity are underdeveloped, whereas in a community project repayment of obligation to other group members may be much stronger (see **box 9**).

BOX 9 Nature of help

To what extent do you agree that...

- Some say that by helping others you help yourself in the long run.
  (Adapted from Bullen and Onyx, 1998)
- People behave in an opportunistic manner and escape their obligations to others whenever they can.
  (Adapted from Sudarsky, 1999)

Antecedents

This element asks why individuals who attend a service or project, chose to participate in the network in the first place. Factors that promote social inclusion are likely to fit this role. Accessibility to transport, distance to the project, health status and time constraints are some examples of pragmatic reasons for attending a group. Assuming participation in the network is a matter of choice and is attainable, these practicalities will be weighed up by the individual against motivations to receive advice, support or new knowledge provided by the relevant network. This issue may be explored by seeking views from people who deliberately choose to forgo membership of the group (see **box 10**).

 © THE SAINSBURY CENTRE FOR MENTAL HEALTH, 2002

BOX 10 Belonging to the group

I don't belong to the support group because:

- It is better to look after oneself.
- We are very spread out
- My needs are too great to be solved by any single group.
- Groups or people like me, do not have people that can help us.
- I've tried before but afterwards the group closed.
- It costs too much effort and there are no concrete results.

(Narayan, 1998)

Consequences

What are the actual advantages of having social capital? This can be looked at in two ways: firstly what are the positive and constructive processes that social capital encourages in a group and secondly what are the consequences of those processes? If optimum antecedents and social capital components are in place then desirable action may result.

Co-operation between individuals, participation by all members, learning of new skills, copying of positive role models and pooling of skills are some general functions that result if the social capital components are maximised (Collier, 1998). The consequences of these functions are less generalisable and depend on the situation.

Co-operation between members of a group, whose objective is to raise funds for a fellow member's hip operation, leads to that member receiving treatment and improving in health and well-being. Co-operation within a football fan club, however, leads to totally different consequences, a lift to the sports ground for example.

Conclusion

It is evident from the above discussion that social capital is a complex idea and that attempting to measure every dimension would be a daunting task. Instead, each evaluation team should choose the dimensions that appear most relevant to the specific context of the evaluation. For example, an emotional support group might prefer to measure the

 © THE SAINSBURY CENTRE FOR MENTAL HEALTH, 2002

development of trust whereas a project whose aim is to unite a neighbourhood and fight crime, may be more interested in the measurement of social cohesion. Whilst focusing upon specific aspects it is important to keep in mind the wider social capital picture in which each component is placed and the possible relationships that may exist between them.

Acknowledgements

The author would like to acknowledge the contributions of Professor Sarah Cowley, Angus Forbes, Jill Maben, Peter Griffiths and Trevor Murrells (Florence Nightingale School of Nursing and Midwifery, King's College London) to the understanding of social capital expressed here. A second acknowledgement is given to the Health Development Agency for the funding received for the exploration of the measurement of social capital.

© THE SAINSBURY CENTRE FOR MENTAL HEALTH, 2002

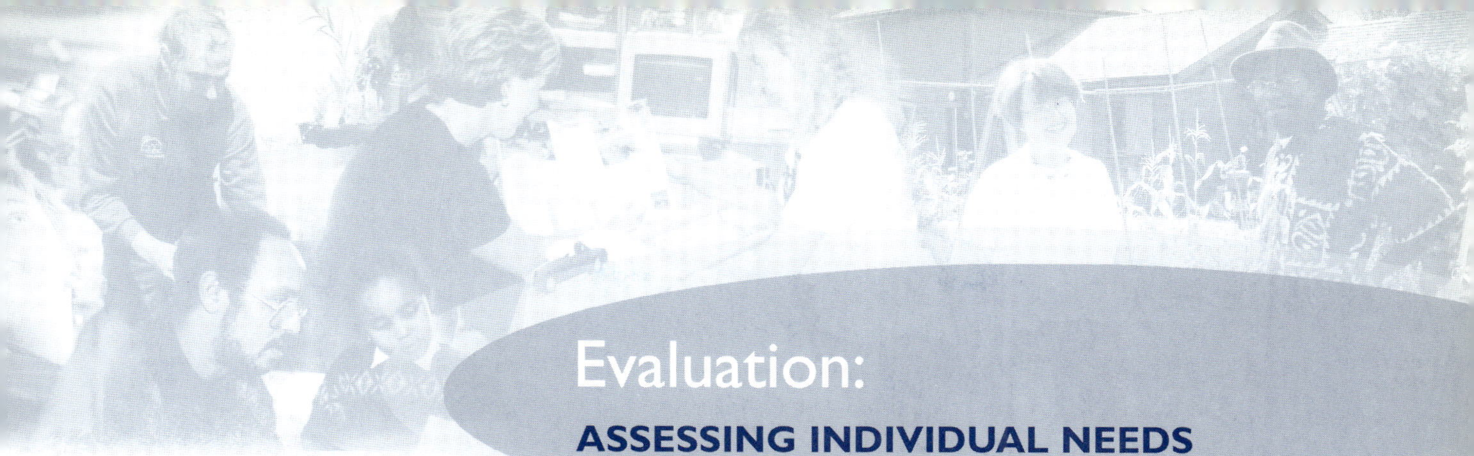

Evaluation:
ASSESSING INDIVIDUAL NEEDS

Fabian A. Davis, Jan Burns, Peter Lindley and Richard K. Sutton

Maintaining assiduous records of a client's life achievements, social involvements, education, work, leisure, housing needs and use of services (including monitoring the number and length of hospital admissions) will show the connection between intervention and outcomes. This rigorous approach to the measurement of client achievement also provides evidence for service planning and can strengthen the case for increased resources. Staff who are willing to engage in data gathering, analysis and interpretation will be open to changing their practices in the light of their findings.

The Support Needs Questionnaire (SNQ) was developed by one of the long-term intervention teams in Oxleas NHS Trust as a way of capturing the information needed for person-centred planning and social inclusion. The questionnaire focuses on the needs of people for support in developing a valued and socially inclusive lifestyle in an 'enabling' rather than 'disablist' framework.

The questionnaire goes through a series of around twenty questions on eight topics: living in your community; getting involved socially; making decisions; being respected and having a role; building on strengths and abilities; money matters; physical health and fitness; and peace of mind. While 160 questions is long for an assessment questionnaire, it provides robust evidence of need and over 200 service users have completed these forms, most preferring to address one topic at a time.

The questions are framed positively to emphasise support for achievement rather than support because of disability, and are mostly about daily activities, the roles, relationships and choices we all make and the skills we all need to fulfil those roles. Added to these items are some questions about the support that might be needed to deal with discrimination or exclusion.

There are also questions on how to ensure good relations with service providers as well as some problem identification items intended to ensure that physical complaints and personal distress do not go unidentified. Service users, their families and independent service user consultants assisted in the choice of items, their wording and the layout of the questionnaire through its various versions over several years.

 © THE SAINSBURY CENTRE FOR MENTAL HEALTH, 2002

The questionnaire has a service user form and a care co-ordinator form and fits easily with the concept and practice of the care programme approach (CPA). It avoids perceiving social inclusion as an optional addition to CPA by reframing the whole CPA process so it becomes the servant of the main goal for mental health services: socially inclusive valued living.

The questionnaire has been evaluated (Davis *et al.*, in press) and has been found to be reliable and valid for people with severe and enduring mental health difficulties. The questionnaire and related materials about person-centred planning have been used extensively in post qualification training at the Sainsbury Centre for Mental Health. Further research on its use is under discussion with assertive outreach teams where their mission is seen as socially inclusive. The current version of the Support Needs Questionnaire is to be published shortly.

Extracts from the care co-ordinator version of the SNQ are shown in **box 1**. Each scale actually consists of twenty items but a selection is shown to give a flavour of the type of issues that are looked at. Requests for reprints/inspection copies of the SNQ should be addressed to Dr Fabian Davis (details on p265).

This article is dedicated to the memory of Richard K. Sutton, user involvement frontiersman, who acted as the user consultant to the research on the SNQ. Richard sadly died before the publication of this resource.

 ©THE SAINSBURY CENTRE FOR MENTAL HEALTH, 2002

BOX 1 Some questions from the support needs questionnaire

Main topic area	Example items	Accomplishment						
	My client would need… ***So they could***	*No help (1)*	*Hardly any help (2)*	*A bit of help (3)*	*A fair amount of help (4)*	*A good deal of help (5)*	*A lot of help (6)*	*A great deal of help (7)*
Living in their neighbourhood – community presence	• Visit their friends/family • Go anywhere without hindrance							
Get involved in their community – community participation	• Join a hobby/interest club • Look after their friends/family							
Making their own decisions – choice	• Decide about their future life • Decide who comes to their CPA							
Having respect and being respected – social roles	• Be someone with a job • Be safe from abuse/prejudice							
Develop to their fullest ability – competence and skills	• Develop a hobby • Look after their sexual health							
Money matters	• Pay their rent/mortgage • Get best value for their money							
	My client ***Needs help with***	*Never (1)*	*Very rarely (2)*	*Rarely (3)*	*Now and then (4)*	*Often (5)*	*Usually (6)*	*Always (7)*
Keeping fit and healthy – physical health	• Eating a balanced diet • Getting enough exercise							
Peace of mind – mental health	• Hearing voices • Having more confidence							

 © THE SAINSBURY CENTRE FOR MENTAL HEALTH, 2002

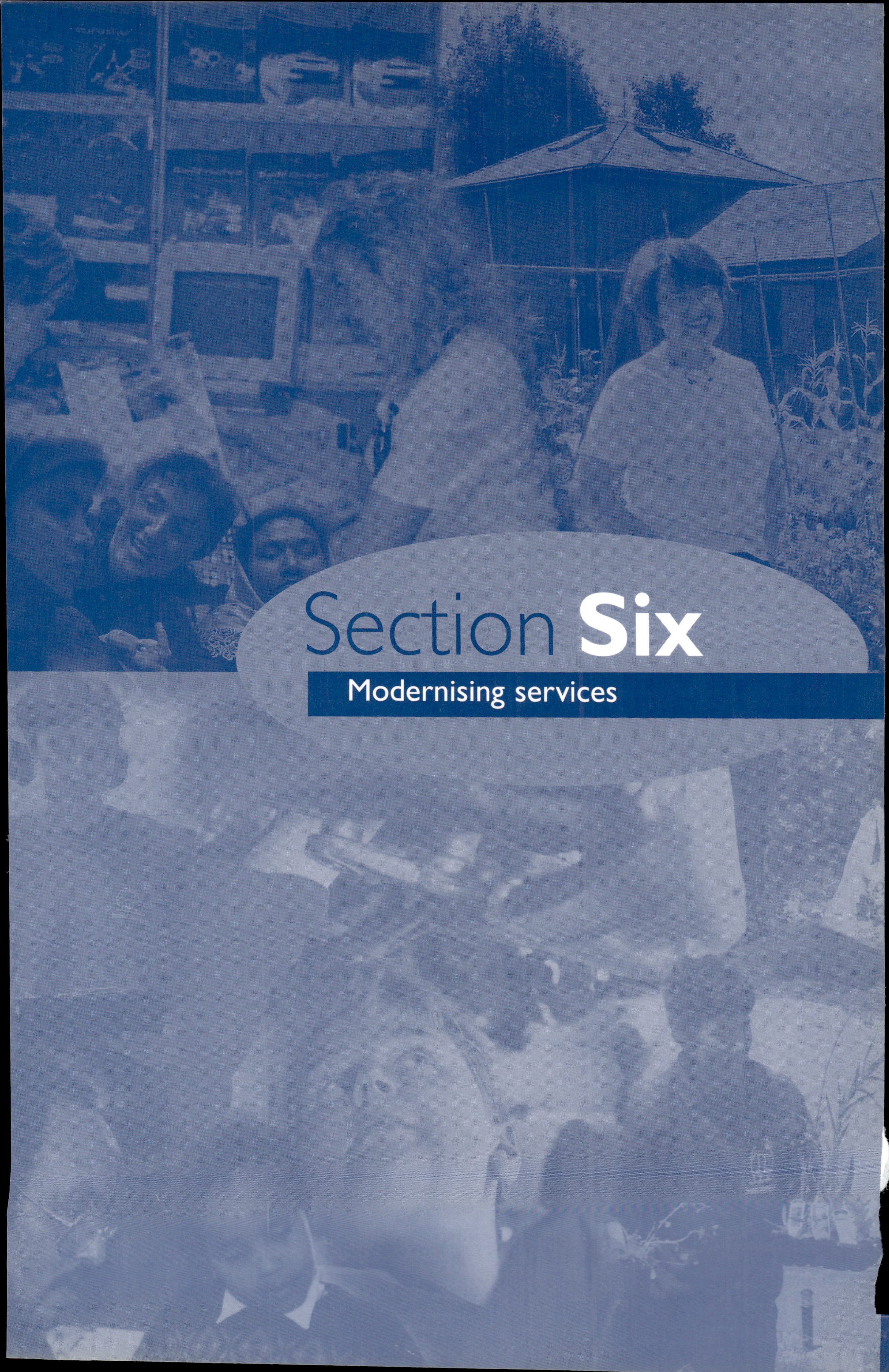

Section Six

Modernising services

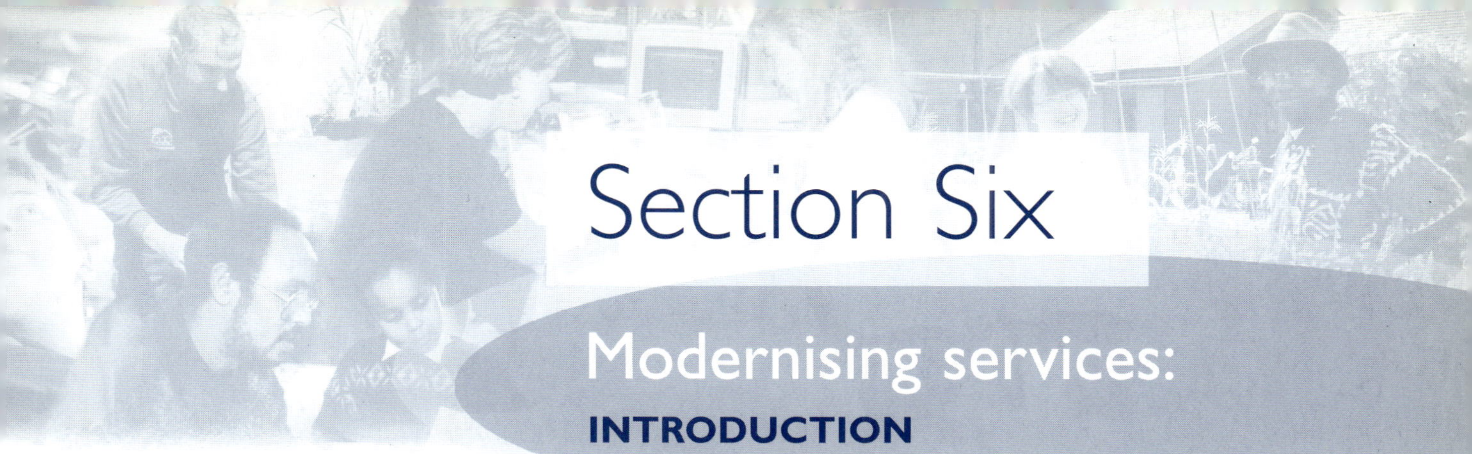

Section Six

Modernising services: INTRODUCTION

Peter Bates

This final section of the book builds on the practical proposals that have been made already and provides some further useful resources to assist both individuals and organisations.

The opening article, *Some Practical Resources,* collects together a few of the practical problems that practitioners have wrestled to solve and proposes working solutions. These are designed to be 'just good enough' to provoke thinking and suggest a way forward, rather than form the last word in user involvement, philosophies, job descriptions, performance and risk management. Many further resources need to be developed in addition to these items, and it is hoped that pioneers will freely share their work to increase the overall toolkit available to new entrants to the field.

Pete Ritchie goes to the heart of the matter when he looks at care planning. The merit of any philosophical and administrative change is shown in the extent to which it yields concrete improvements in quality of life for service users, and Ritchie introduces *Person-centred Planning* as a radical approach to listening and responding to people. While it is easy for anyone to call their approach to assessment and care planning person-centred; we are provided with a sharp description of the approach and its attendant dangers that have been identified over the last 20 years.

Friends, relatives, work colleagues and other associates are drawn into the process of supporting the person, not so much to get a service as to get a life. Ambitions count more than symptoms.

The use of this planning approach with a person who is in crisis may illustrate some of the issues involved. In crisis, one person might assert that their ambition is world domination, while another person might want to die. Person-centred planning works with people who love that person, those who have known them long enough to know their long-term aspirations. For most people, those aspirations include a home, a job, friends and an identity in the community – citizenship and social inclusion.

 © THE SAINSBURY CENTRE FOR MENTAL HEALTH, 2002

But be warned – person-centred planning can seriously damage your traditional bureaucracy! A focus on inclusion will change practice with individuals and change the overarching values and philosophy of mental health and community agencies. This means that the middle of the organisation is under pressure from both sides to adopt practices and procedures that are coherent with the new approach.

Transforming the Whole Organisation sets out the details of this transformation as it affects care management, performance management and strategic management and concludes with a self-evaluation tool to assist in the process of reflection and organisational development.

It is tempting to use the self-evaluation tool within existing decision making settings, such as a senior management team or board. However, part of the challenge is for organisations to think in terms of flatter hierarchies, and wider stakeholder participation with people throughout the organisation and outside it. While inspection processes such as 'best value', 'joint reviews' and 'investors in people' all require that direct care staff and users are consulted before the service review is concluded, a transformed organisation will routinely involve these partners in all its decision making, and not just for the inspection. However it is used, we hope that the self-assessment tool will stimulate reflection, discussion and growth.

Ron Coleman takes us back to basics in the concluding article. Citizenship and social inclusion in mental health is just a fragment of the wider struggle for dignity, recognition and respect shared by many marginalised and oppressed communities.

There is a real danger that inclusion and citizenship will acquire the paraphernalia of a popular movement, with its travelling experts, conference circuit, vociferous adherents and opponents, journals, books and demonstration sites. Meanwhile, the community becomes no more than a new location for the traditional power differences between staff and service users to be played out.

More subtly, while a few people may find that their lives really do improve through access to decent jobs, income and other opportunities, similar rights may still be denied to others such as women who use mental health services, black users, gay and lesbian users, learning disabled users, homeless people, drug users.... Perhaps most pernicious of all, in the development of procedures and outcome measures for inclusion, workers will grow to think that supporting inclusion is a job. Inclusion and citizenship affects us all, 24 hours a day.

 © THE SAINSBURY CENTRE FOR MENTAL HEALTH, 2002

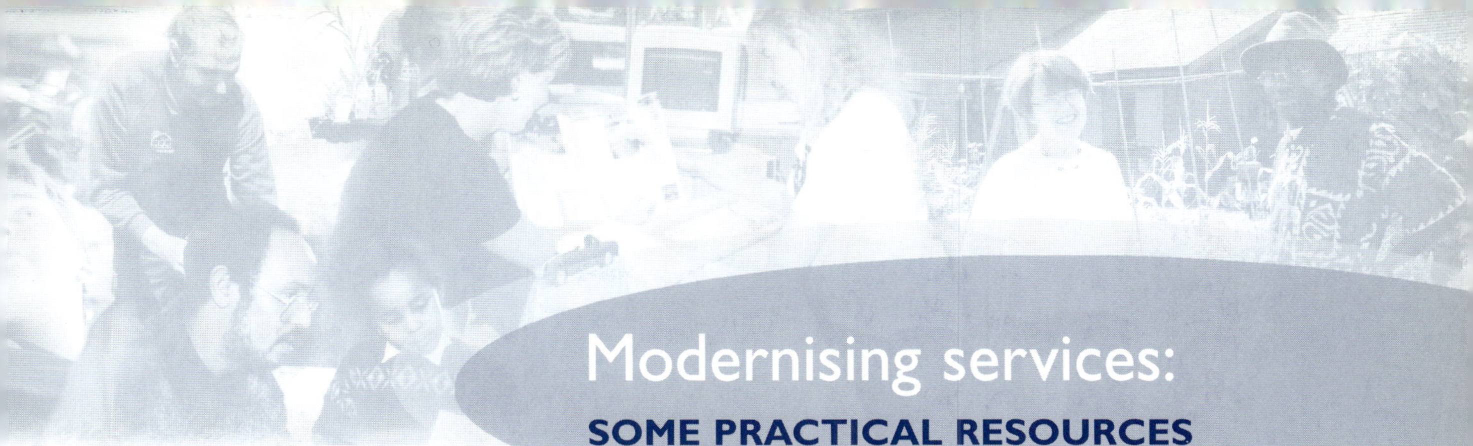

Modernising services:
SOME PRACTICAL RESOURCES

Peter Bates

This section provides a toolbag of resources to help develop inclusive mental health services. It is not a complete set, but may provide some starting points or suggest further work that needs to be done in the future.

Involving service users

Any service that aims to empower people and support them in accessing mainstream opportunities in the wider community will need to take up the challenge of user involvement. Much has been written on this topic elsewhere, and so here we simply provide a few suggestions.

Firstly, an independent advocacy group is an essential component of any user involvement strategy. As will be seen from North Denbighshire (see **box 1**) survivors can control and run the network, set the agenda and take responsibility for stimulating changes in the mental health system. While advocacy groups need to remain independent, the everyday decision making processes within mental health services can be opened out to involve users (see **box 2**).

BOX 1 An independent advocacy group

North Denbighshire Survivors Network

North Denbighshire Survivors Network (NDSN) is open to anyone over the age of 16 years who lives locally and has or has had a mental health problem. Each full member has one vote. Support workers and carers can be associate members but do not have voting rights. The organisation has a management committee and an elected panel of representatives.

Continued overleaf...

 © THE SAINSBURY CENTRE FOR MENTAL HEALTH, 2002

BOX 1 An independent advocacy group/continued…

Funding comes from the health authority and Vale of Clwyd Mind for the purpose of:

- offering mutual support to members;
- providing information exchange;
- enabling members to discuss and voice their views.

Over the past four years, the Network has organised conferences on a wide range of issues ranging from complementary therapies to advocacy.

NDSN members have also attended numerous conferences in Wales and other parts of Britain, contributing to debate and gaining insights and experience to feed back into the support and dissemination activities of the group. Guest speakers at NDSN meetings – which are held twice monthly – have covered topics as diverse as crystal healing and coping with Christmas.

NDSN is an umbrella organisation for:

- a patients' council, held at the Ablett Unit of Glan Clwyd Hospital, Bodelwyddan, near Denbigh;
- a number of other North Denbighshire-based survivor and support groups.

An essential aspect of the ethos of the organisation is that opportunities exist for all members to contribute, but no one is expected to do anything unless they want to.

In conjunction with Vale of Clwyd Mind, NDSN carried out a user-led research project and in 1998 published a document called *In Our View*. The survey focused on service provision, highlighting aspects of good practice and identifying areas where further provision was needed. Copies of this document can be obtained for £1.00 per copy from:

NDSN
34 Elwy Street, Rhyl LL18 1BT
Tel/Fax 01745 354787
Email ndsn@lineone.net

 © THE SAINSBURY CENTRE FOR MENTAL HEALTH, 2002

BOX 2 Involving service users in decision making

- Case records include a clear statement of the service user's opinions.
- Regular community meetings are held where all staff and all users talk together about the service.
- Service users fill in questionnaires about the service.
- An advisory group of service users discuss issues concerning the service.
- The steering group for the service includes service users.
- A group of service users manage their own small budget.
- Service users share decision making about many service budgets.
- Service users hold keys for internal doors or can open buildings out-of-hours.
- Service users participate in maintaining or improving premises.
- Service users are provided with information on how service objectives are met.
- Service users are involved in staff recruitment.
- Service users are paid for specific tasks.

Philosophy of care

The business planning process demands that mental health and other services clarify the principles that lie behind their work. An adequate philosophy statement needs certain elements (see **box 3**).

BOX 3 Components of a comprehensive philosophy of care

Unique contribution

This service provides something unique that would be lost if the team was merged with another or disappeared.

Values and beliefs

This acknowledges the values of the organisation and professional bodies and also identifies the specific values, which define this particular team's work. This may include such values as:

Continued overleaf...

 © THE SAINSBURY CENTRE FOR MENTAL HEALTH, 2002

BOX 3 Components of a comprehensive philosophy of care/continued...

- choice;
- recognising the abilities of the service user;
- the value of roles and relationships in the wider community;
- user empowerment.

Best practice

The team explains in its philosophy how it will learn about successful approaches in other places. Membership of professional associations, access to research journals and similar service providers will feature here.

Success criteria

Precise measures for success are required and the team monitors them on a regular basis taking action to continuously improve the services. Both qualitative and quantitative indicators will feature here, including the accreditation of the skills and learning acquired by service users.

Target clients

Targeting specifies who is to be served from the available population. There is a specific description of how the service is tailored to meet these needs and a specification of the target client group.

Stakeholders

The statement of philosophy needs to show how the team will relate to all the other elements of the organisation and the wider community.

Move-on

Few people stay here forever, so in this section the team explains how it finds out about life beyond the service, identifies skill deficits and specifies what action it takes to help people prepare for moving on.

Wider policy

The team is part of a number of larger structures and so this section of the statement shows how the policy of the team links to organisational and national agendas.

© THE SAINSBURY CENTRE FOR MENTAL HEALTH, 2002

LIBRARY
CHARLES FREARS CAMPUS
DE MONTFORT UNIVERSITY

This philosophy of care was written by a mixed team of service users, staff and other stakeholders (see **box 4**). Several extracts have been selected from a longer document to illustrate how social inclusion can be given real recognition and importance within a mental health service.

BOX 4 Extracts from the philosophy statement of a socially inclusive mental health service

"Positive images should be promoted by developing means of delivering services which are, as much as possible, non-segregationist, non-congregationist, age, gender and culturally appropriate and that follow the routines and rhythms of ordinary society."

"The services should not mark out mentally ill service users by inappropriate associations with other user groups or unfortunate imagery, and should associate people with mental health difficulties with valued members of society in activities, which are of personal and social value. This should be done so people with a mental illness can be seen by the public for their common humanity and increase their opportunities to remain valued members of their communities and to minimise the risks of stigmatisation and discrimination."

"Service users, wherever possible, should be encouraged and supported in their use of resources available to any member of the general public including generic health and social service facilities in addition to places of residence, culture, leisure, education, worship and work. The object of the service is to maintain the client's status and position in society as an ordinary citizen and support their capacity to use non-specialised community facilities and health services including those of the wider health service."

"All efforts at rehabilitation should be first attempted whilst the service user remains in their usual home and daytime environments."

"Where this principle is of necessity to be compromised the rules of thumb: 'use the least restrictive environment' and the 'least socially disruptive (excluding) environment' should be adopted. The length of stay where residential accommodation is required to overcome personal and community challenge should be the shortest possible and be as near to home as possible. The service should actively support social continuity wherever possible. No service user should be placed in any form of accommodation away from home without commitment to a plan designed to enable them to return as soon as possible."

Continued overleaf...

BOX 4 Extracts from the philosophy statement of a socially inclusive mental health service/continued...

"The service should support the integration of specialist provisions into local communities by advocating for the placing of mental health facilities together with ordinary facilities meeting the same kind of basic need. For example, a housing scheme should be in the heart of a well-populated, well thought of and safe residential area and a work scheme should be at the heart of a working area or industrial complex of good repute. These matters are essential prerequisites for a service that is serious about promoting social integration in as ordinary a setting as possible."

"The service should actively debate the dilemmas inherent in its task. The service should develop an atmosphere of tolerance and provide active support to staff who work with the uncertainty those dilemmas evoke everyday in order to support the often slow, but necessarily progressive improvement in service users' mental state and their capacity for ordinary living." (Dr Fabian A. Davis)

Job descriptions

Few job descriptions give priority to social inclusion or specify exactly what is required in terms of providing support for people to participate in community life. The job description set out in **box 5** is an attempt to be specific about the duties that promote social inclusion. Some individual workers might adopt this description in its entirety, while others would add additional responsibilities, or delete some elements as they are covered elsewhere in the agency.

BOX 5 A job description

Job summary

- To develop access routes into a range of activities in the ordinary community alongside other members of the public.

Duties

- To demonstrate an understanding of people with mental health problems, particularly as this relates to access to community inclusion. To support people with mental health problems in making informed choices about their own community participation. To negotiate opportunities for people with mental health problems to participate in community life.

Continued opposite...

BOX 5 A job description/continued...

- To demonstrate experience and knowledge of a wide range of opportunities in the community. To be responsible for the compilation of an up-to-date database of opportunities available in the community. This involves detailed research and networking into the statutory, voluntary and commercial sector. It includes specific searches for resources which are targeted at minority and under-represented groups.
- To advertise and market information about current opportunities for community participation to service users. Material will be presented to users and staff in an attractive and accessible manner.
- To build partnerships with other community agencies so as to foster understanding, access resources and create a wide spectrum of opportunities for people with mental health problems. This will include identifying, challenging and working with fear or prejudice about mental illness. The worker will promote awareness of users' rights to access all services and provide support to the agency to facilitate successful placements. Support may include encouraging agencies to develop new arrangements.
- To demonstrate good communication skills with users, staff and agencies in the community and an ability to work across agencies which may have different aims and value systems. To ensure that ongoing support is available for service users and community organisations.
- To utilise a thorough knowledge of how to become involved in community groups and how relationships are built and maintained. In consultation with others at the placement site and elsewhere, to review the progress that service users make in the placement environment.
- To work directly with identified individuals in community settings, supporting the person to participate to a maximum extent as a full and equal member of the setting.
- To provide support to people in the host agency in order to facilitate successful placement.
- To work as part of the team and be creative, flexible, innovative, tenacious and supportive. To work flexible hours in order to achieve the team's objectives.

 © THE SAINSBURY CENTRE FOR MENTAL HEALTH, 2002

Performance management

A checklist of performance areas for a team that is promoting community-based opportunities for people with mental health problems is set out in **box 6**. Each area can be converted into a specific indicator and performance target that is appropriate for the individual service.

BOX 6 Performance

Getting the message across

- Publicity events are frequent in both mental health and community venues, written materials are available in day centres and other places where service users may attend, and referral agents have accurate information about opportunities.

Is the project serving the right people?

- The population served is representative of the wider population of the area.
- Referrals accepted by age, gender and ethnicity are comparable with reference data on the wider population of mental health service users.
- The project works with people who have serious mental health difficulties.
- The project works with people who have had a long career in mental health services (since contact with mental health services gradually erodes social roles and networks).

Does the project work?

- Host organisations (employers, colleges, leisure activity providers etc. who include people with mental health problems) tell us about (i) changes they have made to their service as a result of user and staff involvement; (ii) their level of satisfaction with the support they have received from the mental health service.
- Intervention by the project increases social roles and relationships for people who want this.
- Service users like the project.

Managing risk

Material on the assessment and management of risk is common, but rather less is available on the implications of a socially inclusive approach. Risks can include: health and safety hazards; a dissatisfying activity can lead to an individual feeling bored or stressed; distress or violent behaviour can lead to a person harming themselves, other people or property;

and the denial of an opportunity means that they may fail to reach their potential. Risks can arise at the community site and elsewhere.

From a social inclusion perspective, one might assert that behaviour in health and social care settings can be a poor predictor of behaviour in other places; that past behaviour is not always a predictor of future behaviour, and that professionals are often overly pessimistic about the abilities of their clients.

Where community agencies receive problem-focused information from health and social care staff there is a danger that this will erode their expectations and optimism for the person, leading to a downward spiral of deteriorating behaviour and further reductions in optimism.

In consequence, some staff are eager to provide opportunities for someone to gain a fresh start and leave behind any negative reputation that may have accrued in the health and social care setting. Within this framework, risk assessment is carried out on the basis of certain assumptions (see **box 7**).

BOX 7 Risk values

- The individual has the potential to be the best judge of risk, rather than other people. For this to work he or she must be provided with good information about the environment and her/his views and preferences must be taken very seriously within a context of empowerment.
- The individual's history belongs first to them and is not the property of professionals.
- Current feelings, opinions and behaviour are more important than past events.
- Risk is an intimate subject that is shy of power imbalances and so it can only be discussed sensibly in the context of mutual, trusting relationships. This makes it important to build relationships rather than demand that a 'disclosure consent' form is signed before resources are released.
- A satisfying lifestyle is a right and may lead to the reduction of risk, rather than enjoyable opportunities being used as a reward for behaving well and safely.

 © THE SAINSBURY CENTRE FOR MENTAL HEALTH, 2002

These beliefs lead to a risk management strategy that pays attention to the following things (see **box 8**).

BOX 8 Risk strategy

An inclusive risk strategy will:

- assess environments and procedures to ensure that risks are minimised;
- recognise that people and environments are unique and so arrangements must be tailored to the person in that setting, rather than expecting a single 'risk assessment form' to cover all situations;
- empower the person – a confident and assertive person is more likely to speak up if he or she feels unsafe;
- provide good information about community opportunities. As well as providing good information about the setting itself, information about the procedures that are used in that setting may lead some people to choose an alternative environment in order to avoid the process. For example, explaining the process for checking criminal records prior to work with children might lead someone to choose a different activity;
- train everyone in health and safety, food hygiene and/or dealing with aggression, so that risk becomes a public issue and everyone can share responsibility for keeping each other safe;
- establish a strong relationship between the person and support staff;
- remember that the specific setting in which a person is included can provide some safeguards, in that there are usually other people around who have a range of different kinds of relationships with one another and those in charge. It may be easier to speak out in this kind of setting than it would be in a place where everyone is within the same hierarchy, such as a hospital or residential care establishment.

Conclusion

This section has included a few basic tools that we hope will assist in the journey towards a more inclusive mental health service. There are many other tools that have not been explained here, such as negotiating the specifics of confidentiality and disclosure, cross agency support and mentoring, and the range of available strategies for the support of individuals.

Some of these tools have been invented some time ago and used safely and effectively for years in a quiet corner, while others need to be created and tested out. There is a great deal more work to do, both in disseminating good practice and developing new approaches.

 © THE SAINSBURY CENTRE FOR MENTAL HEALTH, 2002

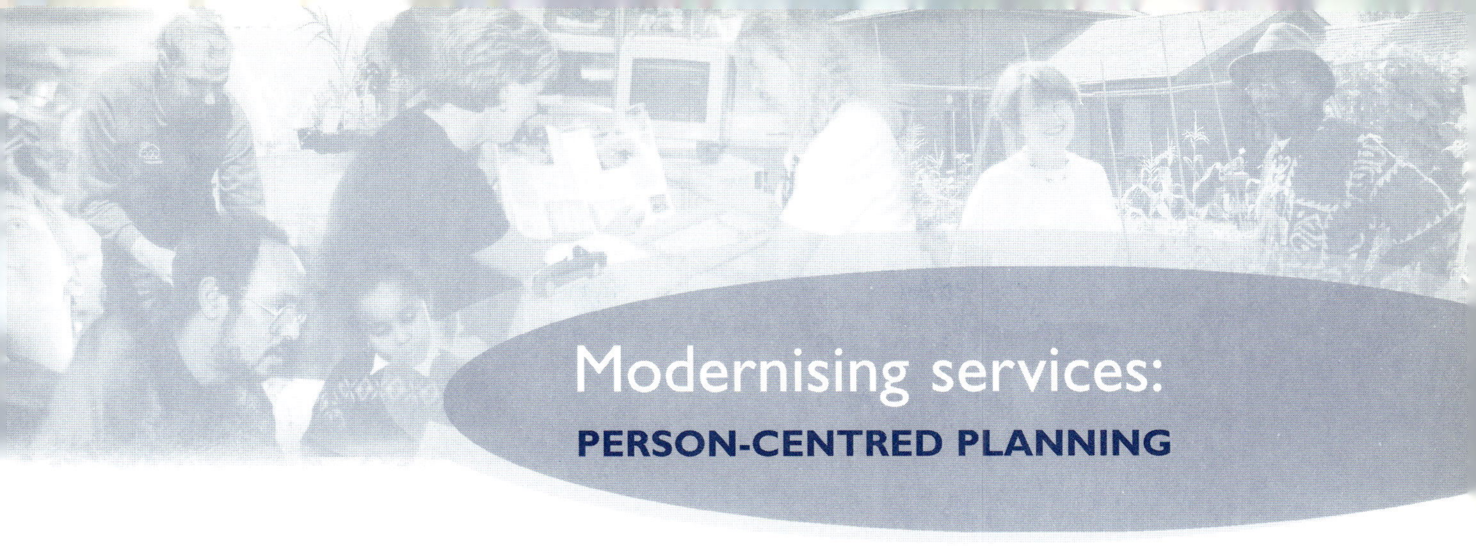

Modernising services:
PERSON-CENTRED PLANNING

Pete Ritchie

Person-centred planning is a way of organising around one person to define and create a better future. This way of working has evolved over the last twenty years, mainly in the US and the UK. Thousands of people and families have used person-centred planning to help them make decisions and changes in their lives.

Typically in person-centred planning an individual invites people who know and like them to come to a meeting. One or two facilitators guide and record the discussions and decisions. After the meeting, people do what's been agreed.

This hardly sounds revolutionary. But the frame which is put around the meeting, the questions the meeting asks, and the way the meeting is organised, often mean that new possibilities emerge, new understandings develop, new alliances are formed and people's lives take a definite turn for the better.

The defining features of person-centred planning

Person-centred planning is a philosophy and an approach, not just a set of tools and techniques. However, the family of tools that are used in person-centred planning provide a practical demonstration of philosophy in action.

Person-centred planning has evolved as a philosophy, a method and a craft over the last 20 years. Key figures in this evolution include Marsha Forest, Susan Burke-Harrison, Herb Lovett, Connie Lyle O'Brien, Beth Mount, John O'Brien, Jack Pearpoint, Michael Smull, Judith Snow and Jack Yates. David Sibbet's work on group graphics (Sibbet, 1981) was also an important influence.

For a definitive account of the evolution of person-centred planning, see O'Brien and Lyle O'Brien (2000). For an overview of person-centred planning, *"its limitations, conditions for success, and contribution to organisational renewal"*, see O'Brien and Lyle O'Brien (1999). Sanderson *et al.*, (1997) provide a full account of how the different tools have been applied in a UK context.

 © THE SAINSBURY CENTRE FOR MENTAL HEALTH, 2002

Person-centred planning tools share an underlying structure (see **box 1**).

BOX 1 Person-centred planning

Asking different questions	Inviting contribution	Recognising urgency – what if nothing changes?	Enrolling	Generating options
SYNTHESIS	*Gathering insights and intelligence*	*Making a judgement about fit*	*Making a commitment to change*	*Planning what to do*
Using the person's language Checking out and checking back	Affirming gifts and capacities	Imagining alternatives Clarifying values	Owning authority	Sharing responsibility

They also share the following features:

Steeped in values

Person-centred planning grew out of a commitment to inclusion as a social goal and was consciously designed as an inclusive process. There is a fundamental coherence between the goal – what person-centred planning is helping people to achieve; and the process – how person-centred planning works.

For example:

- We think that there are people out there who are willing to help in new ways if we ask them properly – so person-centred planning invites contribution from the people present at the meeting.
- We think that many disabled people experience a lack of control in their lives and feel they are managed by the service system rather than managing their services. So person-centred planning gives people as much control and direction as possible – over who comes to the meeting, when and where it is and how long it lasts.
- We think that many disabled people live in enforced absence from communities – so person-centred planning makes sure they are present.

© THE SAINSBURY CENTRE FOR MENTAL HEALTH, 2002

- We think that many people labelled disabled have gifts and capacities that go unnoticed and unused in our communities, so person-centred planning draws attention to people's gifts and capacities and takes these as the starting-point.
- We think that what happens to people labelled disabled is powerfully shaped by mental models: the person's sense of her own identity, and how she and the people around her see each other and understand the part they play in each other's lives. So person-centred planning asks: "Who is this person?" and offers a space for the person to assert a new identity and for others both to affirm this identity and confirm their investment in it. Person-centred planning invites people to enlarge their understanding of the person and to see them through different lenses. As they do this, they also reconsider their own place in the person's world.

Accountability to the person

Person-centred planning is an event in the person's life, not a procedure of the service system. As much as possible, it takes place in the person's world, with the service system seen as part of the environment. The facilitator is accountable to the person who is the focus of the plan. Jo's meeting is Jo's meeting.

The tools and techniques of person-centred planning can be used to manipulate the person into compliance with the service system or with powerful others. However, this is not person-centred planning, any more than sawing up firewood is carpentry.

A commitment to action

While an assessment can stand alone as a description of the person and her situation, a planning process without a commitment to action is unfinished.

Focus on the whole person

Traditional assessment starts from a 'categoric' perspective. The frame around the assessment is the question: "What do people who have this diagnosis typically need?" The discussion is steeped in assumptions about 'people like Jo' – that they belong with 'people like them', that other people will find them a burden, that they don't know their own mind. In this sort of discussion, people are not seeing Jo at all, just her diagnosis.

In a more individualised approach to assessment, people do focus down on Jo and try to set aside the 'group' frame. However, they focus on Jo's disability – what Jo can't do, what's wrong with Jo and what would make Jo better. This makes sense, because disability is what

 © THE SAINSBURY CENTRE FOR MENTAL HEALTH, 2002

the different professionals and agencies have in common. Being an expert in disability qualifies someone to participate in the assessment.

Person-centred planning, though, is about Jo and not about Jo's disability. Jo's disability is acknowledged and respected as one of her identities – but the focus of the plan is on Jo's aspirations, what Jo longs to do; on her preferences, what Jo loves to do; on her relationships, who Jo needs to see; and on her contribution, what Jo – the unique, multi-faceted Jo – can offer the world.

The planning focuses on how Jo can use her gifts to connect with others, not on how Jo can be fixed. The planning starts from the assumption that Jo is OK, that she is just fine as she is. This doesn't mean she doesn't need help, in fact she might die in 12 hours without help, or that it wouldn't be helpful for her to learn some new things if she wants to change things in her life. But Jo is already a whole person, not a part person.

Unique events

Although all person-centred planning shares a common architecture, every planning event is different. All four elements of the planning process are interactive exchanges, and the planning is what happens during and after these exchanges. What happens depends on who is there at the time, and what happens will be different next time.

Each meeting is consciously planned – where should it be, who is invited by whom, how will we use the space, what sequence of questions might work – and is under continuous review – are we getting stuck, are we staying focused on what matters to the person, are the right people being heard, what is not being said. By contrast, care planning meetings often follow a standard format and have a similar feel even when significant people are absent or when one person from an agency has substituted for another.

The graphic record is the planning's footprint – the evidence that planning passed this way. The real plan is not in the paper but in what people do next. Person-centred planning is an event, not a document. By contrast, an assessment is given objective status as a document and can be discussed and passed on independently of the person or of anyone involved in producing it.

© THE SAINSBURY CENTRE FOR MENTAL HEALTH, 2002

Facilitation

Person-centred planning relies on facilitation to move the energy in a situation to a more productive state. There can be many reasons why the energy in and around the person is not being well used.

For example, the individual may not be allowed to shape her own future or even to know what is being planned. Sometimes, families and friends are not involved at all, or are told only what someone else thinks they should hear, or their views and their contributions are discounted even before they are heard.

Sometimes, the professionals around the individual are working in parallel or at cross-purposes, and sometimes this continues even when people know it is happening. Sometimes, people's perception of who the individual is constricts their imagination about what might be possible, and often people start from the service solution end: "Have we got a place for Jo?" and are stuck because there are no slots to slot Jo into. But most of all, the energy is poorly used because people are not thinking about Jo.

Facilitation is a skilful process of realigning the energy around Jo and Jo's aspirations – eliciting, confirming, relating, summarising, re-presenting, questioning, inviting, reflecting, focusing, pushing, encouraging, interpreting, checking out.

It is difficult to facilitate a plan when you have a close interest in what happens afterwards or when you are a part of how things got to be the way they are. Your own hopes and fears for the future or your own defensiveness about the past are noisy and stop you hearing other voices. Some people might imagine that if an individual facilitates her own plan he or she will have more choice, control and status, but the reverse is true. Having a facilitator to help you plan is like having someone cut your hair – they can see all the way round.

Gerry Smale and colleagues describe three models of assessment: the questioning model, the procedural model and the exchange model (Smale, 1993). In the questioning model, the professional's role is to apply her professional expertise to the situation to determine the correct 'diagnosis' and asks questions from that perspective. In the procedural model, the professional is also very much in control of the process, but her starting-point is her administrative authority to allocate resources.

In the exchange model *"it is assumed that all people are expert in their own problems and that there is no reason to assume that the worker will or should ever know more about people and their problems than they do themselves, and certainly not before they do"* (Smale, 1993). The professional's authority derives from his or her skill in facilitating and negotiating exchange between the people involved in the situation. Person-centred planning is firmly within the exchange model.

 © THE SAINSBURY CENTRE FOR MENTAL HEALTH, 2002

Exchange is a source of energy and insight. When people with different perspectives and different requirements engage in dialogue, new understandings can emerge and new solutions can be generated to problems. Equally, if only half the stakeholders are present, consensus may be more easily achieved but the hard work of engaging with difference has only been postponed. As far as possible, person-centred planning puts 'the whole system in the room' and works with the difference.

Facilitators use marginality – being on the boundary – to assist people to exchange. They dance on the edge between the person and the people close to her. They dance on the edge between the 'ordinary' world of the person and her family and the 'special' world of services and professionals. They belong in neither world. If they lean too far towards persuasion or coercion they lose their authority.

However, facilitators are not neutral. They believe that abuse and neglect are wrong, that people's civil and human rights should be upheld, that people should flourish and not just exist. They are biased towards inclusion.

Use of graphics

Person-centred planning typically uses graphic facilitation. In very small meetings, the back of an envelope will do, but when there are more than two or three people a large sheet of wallpaper works better. A graphic has a distinctive power, which has nothing to do with people's ability to read.

The graphic:

- creates a focus of attention for the whole group – people watch the paper, not each other;
- confirms that people have been heard. People who are used to not being heard soon see that their words become real when they go on the paper. If people think the facilitator missed or misunderstood what they said, they can point this out and see it being corrected then and there;
- conveys emotion and vibrancy through colour and shape and size and helps to keep depth and richness in the room. It stores energy and makes it available throughout the meeting;
- shows the relationship between one issue and another. A traditional written report has only one dimension – words go before or after other words. A graphic has two dimensions so it is easier to see patterns.
- helps the facilitators to recap from time to time, pointing to what people have said;
- is unique – and is handed to the person at the end as a shared version of events.

 © THE SAINSBURY CENTRE FOR MENTAL HEALTH, 2002

Because the graphic uses shape and colour and position and icons as well as text, when people go back and look at the graphic, it is much easier to remember the meeting and who said what than when people go through a written minute.

Asking different questions, using different language

Person-centred planning asks different questions, because it is interested in getting to a different place. Each question has a rationale, and the phrasing of each question is considered carefully, for example:

- **What's the story?**

This simple question is deeply layered. The story is what people choose to tell, there and then on the day. The story is also the dominant account of who the person is – an account that the person may or may not accept and which may or may not be deeply damaging. The story is both more than and less than 'Jo's story'.

- **What's the dream?**

Allowing and helping people to dream unlocks the present. Most people do not know what their dream is until they tell it to others. Having your dream heard and respected generates a feeling of safety, often for the first time. The dream is a source of energy, and contains the seeds for what to do next.

- **What's the nightmare?**

For many people, running away from the nightmare is a more powerful force than working towards the dream. So naming the nightmare and bringing it out into the shared daylight can be hugely liberating.

- **What brings out the best in Jo?**

This beautiful question gets people to think carefully and positively about Jo in relation to others; about Jo as a person who is different in different environments; about how to work with what works for Jo. And while Jo knows some of the answers already, she doesn't know them all, and the conversation helps everyone get a clearer understanding.

Key points

- Find someone to (a) review the literature, and (b) attend training on person-centred planning.
- It is easy to claim that your work is 'client-centred' or 'person-centred'. Is anyone using person-centred planning in your locality?

© THE SAINSBURY CENTRE FOR MENTAL HEALTH, 2002

Case Study Person-centred planning in practice: opportunities and dangers

John is a man in his 40s who lives near Edinburgh. He currently lives on his own with support from Connect Housing Association. His parents live a few miles away and they have all just gone on holiday together to Cyprus. John is a part-time college student and is learning to use computers. Most evenings he visits a couple of close friends who live locally and they often play pool. John is currently looking for work either as a cook or a gardener.

For many years John lived in a privately managed small hostel for people with mental health problems. He had to fit in with the other six people. Bed was at 9.30pm; lights out at 10.00pm. He went to a mental health day centre during the week. At the weekend he only got out for half an hour. The social worker used to come to see him and ask how he was getting on. John would say: *"I'm not coping"* and she would say: *"You'll just have to grin and bear it."*

John was referred to Connect Housing when the manager of the private hostel retired. He moved into a shared house managed by the housing association and around the same time he got a new social worker. John was invited to use person-centred planning to think about his future and how he wanted to lead his life.

Before the meeting John chose a few people who knew him well and, with one of the facilitators for the plan, went to ask them some questions – questions like: *"What do you admire about John?"* and: *"What makes a good day for John?"*

John invited various people to come to the first meeting – his parents, his social worker, someone from the day centre, someone from the housing association and a couple of friends. They met in the housing association office and used a large sheet of 'wallpaper' to record the discussion and the decisions. As John says:

> *"It was a bit strange. People were saying good things about me. I managed to get through it all. Dad came out with a lot of good things. It was a blank sheet before we put pen and paper to it. What came out of it? A lot. My past is my past – let's look forward. My future holds a lot this year."*

Since then, John has moved to his own house; stopped going to the day centre; taken a college course; established some close friendships with people living locally; taught a friend to play pool; learned to manage everyday tasks like cooking stir fries and doing the ironing; and worked out some coping strategies for the ups and downs (*"I've been going in even if I feel miserable – I never skip art."*).

The group has kept meeting every few months to help John take stock and plan ahead:

> *"I look forward to these meetings... when they're finished I'm glad to get home. We've had about four meetings, everything's come out positive. Every time it came round I got more confidence about dealing with the bad things."*

What's different about person-centred planning?

- Different people come – John's friends and family are equal contributors in the meetings, alongside professionals. As John says: *"This was the first time they've felt involved. Before then it was just decisions made."*
- People come by invitation – it's up to John to say who he wants at the meeting and nobody has an automatic right to be there. John in turn has been invited to help a friend with his plan.
- There's a different style – the facilitators keep the meeting focused on helping John work out what he wants to do and how he wants to go about it. The meetings are positive and lively, and the graphic recording helps to track and summarise the discussion.
- Everyone is involved in follow-up work after the meeting – John's task last time was to sort out getting a computer and setting it up.
- The meeting asks different questions. John's negative reputation preceded him to the housing association. It would have been easy to focus on John's problems and on how to 'fix' John or where to 'place' him. Person-centred planning focused instead on John's gifts and capacities and on where he wanted to go with his life.
- There is a very practical respect for John's preferences. John said he wanted to live on his own. He says: *"My parents weren't quite sure. Now my Dad comes on a Sunday, helps with the grass cutting. He's taught me to play golf."*
- John said he wanted his own garden, and this is now an important part of his life.
- John did a person specification for his support worker. *"I wanted someone nice, kind, my age who was good at pool (but now I've found someone else to play with) who isn't bossy and is good at listening"* – and then used this as the basis for interviewing and choosing Linda.
- Person-centred planning is not about doing things to John or for John – but nor is it about saying: *"Here you go, John, you're on your own now, you can do everything yourself".* It's about people who know and like John doing things **with** John, and recognising that John – like all of us – needs other people's support to be his own person.
- He says: *"Living on my own is perfect... I can do what I want, come home when I feel like it... it's my weekend."*

© THE SAINSBURY CENTRE FOR MENTAL HEALTH, 2002

Better and worse ways of using person-centred planning

Like every innovation, person-centred planning has its champions and its critics. It will deliver more than its detractors wish and less than its enthusiasts claim. A thoughtful person – wherever they stand in the mental health world – will go back a stage before deciding how best to use this approach, and will ask:

What is the problem person-centred planning is designed to solve?

Person-centred planning is designed to overcome inertia – the tendency for things to continue in a straight line. For many disabled people, the status quo is isolation, invisibility, and dependence. Others define their identity, they live to other people's clocks, and their life is restricted by the absence of their own power or by the misuse of other people's power.

Many people are detained – often kindly – in 'serviceland' – both in the old serviceland, physically behind the wall, and in the new serviceland, physically in and among the real world but subtly separate, out of phase, never quite connecting to the ordinary.

Wolfensberger and Glenn (1975) asked the question: *"What are the likely consequences for this person if current practice does not change?"* For many people the answer is 'more of the same' – left to itself, the current situation will not generate change. Person-centred planning focuses energy around the person so they can choose a different path. Sometimes inertia is too strong and the best planning in the world is unable to deflect the forces constraining the person's life. Sometimes there is plenty of room to work and only a light touch is needed to chart a new direction.

If this is the purpose for which person-centred planning is designed, a thoughtful person would quickly see the dangers of seeking to assimilate person-centred planning into the service system. Even their best friends would admit that service systems are experts in inertia – at keeping on keeping on.

Danger one: the belief that services are what people need most

The inspirational nature of person-centred planning takes it outside the context of service planning; much of what people need and want is not available within the mental health service system. Person-centred planning does not demand that the service system provides these things; rather it acknowledges the limitations of the service system and invites people to engage with the person in working for what they want outside the system.

 © THE SAINSBURY CENTRE FOR MENTAL HEALTH, 2002

Danger two: having no power to act when change is called for

People can learn to use the tools and apply the techniques of person-centred planning within a context where all people are going to be allowed to have is what they have already got; and service workers who have promoted person-centred planning in good faith find that they cannot honour their commitments. Unless the system is willing to disinvest and reinvest, at least at the margins, then person-centred planning from within the service system will lead to cynicism.

Danger three: cut-down versions

The leading practitioners in person-centred planning have been learning for over twenty years. It is entirely possible to take their work, strip out the philosophy, ignore the underlying theory, dull the edge of their questions, forgo their commitment to uniqueness, confuse their purpose and discount their dilemmas.

It is easy to make a thin, shiny thing and call it person-centred planning and produce computer templates for people's plans. This proceduralisation starkly relocates person-centred planning within the administrative nexus: we can generate your plan from our template. These attenuated versions of person-centred planning may cause a slight rash for a few days but will certainly inoculate the system against the real thing.

Danger four: expecting person-centred planning to do the system's work

It doesn't need person-centred planning to see that services are letting people down. Making services more responsive and relevant; freeing up money so that people get direct control over the services they use; having professionals on tap not on top; confronting poor quality – none of these depend on person-centred planning. There is a danger of systems postponing reform until they have finished doing their person-centred plans.

Danger five: covering up some or all of the other dangers

The real danger is when people refuse to look at what is really happening.

© THE SAINSBURY CENTRE FOR MENTAL HEALTH, 2002

So, what's a better way of using person-centred planning?

First, recognise that the system needs its own systems, and that person-centred planning should remain marginal to these. Aim for person-centred thinking to infect rather than inoculate the system, but don't try to build in or mandate person-centred planning as a specific process.

Second, invest in developing a community of practice over time. Invest in initial learning, do a few plans well. Recruit people with natural talent as facilitators from different backgrounds and give them time to become skilled and discerning. Encourage people engaged in person-centred planning to meet, reflect and write.

Third, get commissioners to listen to people who have had plans and to facilitators who have been planning with people. See what the patterns are and think about how the system could flex a little.

 © THE SAINSBURY CENTRE FOR MENTAL HEALTH, 2002

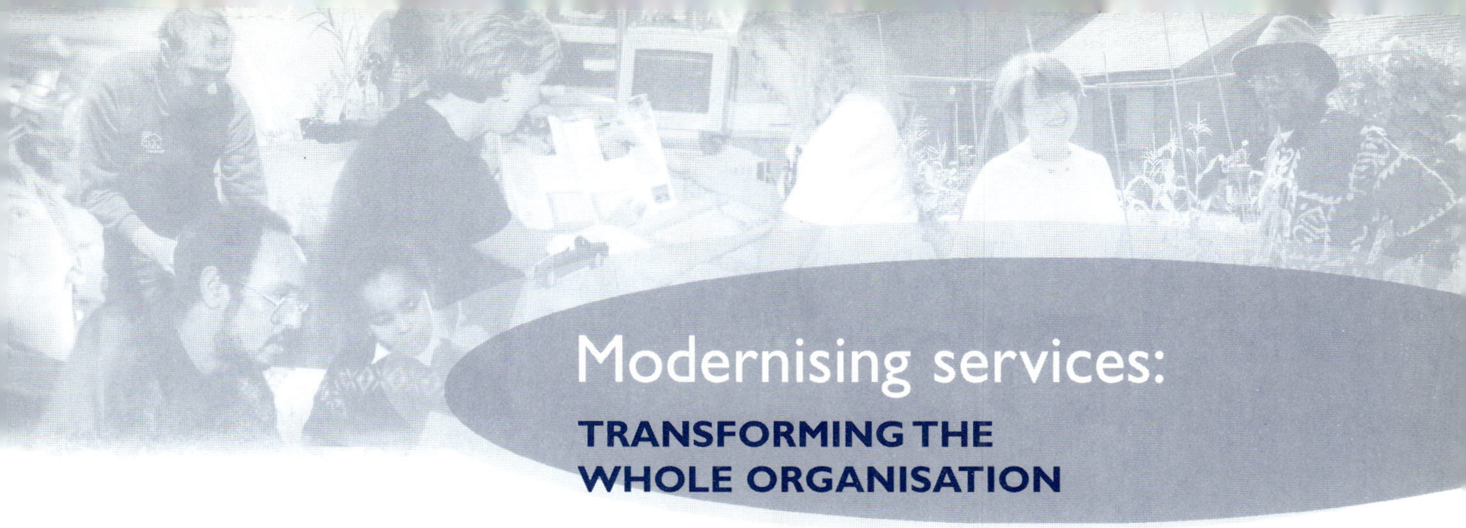

Modernising services:

TRANSFORMING THE WHOLE ORGANISATION

Peter Bates, Clive Miller and Paul Taylor

In this article, we outline the defining characteristics of an inclusive organisation and suggest how these characteristics link with existing policy imperatives.

Inclusive organisations

Unless the whole organisation is geared up to inclusion, inclusive services and outcomes cannot be sustained. While direct care staff can support service users to establish an included life, other employees within the agency have to play their part as well. This approach – beginning with the outcomes that service users desire and working backwards to redesign the organisation – is a common feature of inclusive approaches.

However, many of these approaches only lightly sketch in the organisational requirements to support inclusive services, paying most attention to how to organise front line management and service delivery teams. We take this thinking a stage further by exploring in greater detail the inclusive requirements at four levels of the organisation – care management, performance management, resource management and strategic management.

We chose these four aspects because they are the core areas on which *Joint Reviews of Social Services* focus when indicating the types of improvements necessary to develop and sustain effective front line practice.

A best value approach begins by identifying the outcomes that service users and local people value. It then questions whether the current range of services and the way they are delivered is the most effective way of securing those outcomes within the available resources. Similarly, management, planning and quality assurance processes are then evaluated to establish whether they provide the best way of supporting the delivery of those services and making them accountable to service users and local people.

As the *Joint Reviews* (Audit Commission, 1998; Audit Commission, 1999) stress, these characteristics are not discrete. Here they serve as magnets to gather and order the array of features that have to change when an organisation moves towards social inclusion.

 © THE SAINSBURY CENTRE FOR MENTAL HEALTH, 2002

Some of the features we discuss have already been identified as good practice by the joint reviews while others take the practice a stage further.

Care management

We need to begin by challenging this term, as an inclusive organisation will be more focused upon service user's ambitions than their assessed needs. Of course there are times when users genuinely want things that will harm themselves or others, and the government is taking steps to increase protection of both service users and the wider community (Home Office and Department of Health, 1999; Department of Health and Home Office, 2000).

It is our contention that these times are relatively infrequent within the whole spectrum of support, but have enjoyed a disproportionate influence over the culture of the mental health services and led to paternalism. This over-emphasis upon control has favoured diagnosis by professionals over personal growth; needs assessment over personal goal setting; and treatment compliance over a personal journey of recovery.

An inclusive organisation will listen very carefully to the goals and ambitions of service users and will expend energy in helping people achieve their own life goals. A variety of surveys have shown that most service users will ask for a decent home, education, employment, satisfying leisure time and positive relationships with a diverse group of other citizens (Faulkner and Layzell, 2000; Rose, 2001).

Hence users should be enabled to set out what kind of support they need to achieve these goals. This will inevitably mean that professional services will have to take their place alongside other, informal sources of support – from relatives, friends and co-participants in a variety of community settings.

Meetings to review progress will often take place in the evening or at the weekend and will happen in clients' homes, not clinics. Regular monitoring of client records will show that support plans tend to be unique, are relevant to the personal goals of service users, targets are achieved and the plan is regularly updated.

Service users will find that an increasing proportion of their life is conducted outside health and social care settings, alongside and in relationship with people who are not paid to provide therapeutic inputs to the individual. Leisure activities outside of office hours will be supported as well as activity in traditional working hours.

The service user will be able to look back and trace a recovery pathway and identify the things that have helped or hindered (Deegan, 1996). The present will consist of effective support to engage in a valued life in the community and a feeling of being part of things

 © THE SAINSBURY CENTRE FOR MENTAL HEALTH, 2002

rather than isolated and bored. Ambitions for the future will be in sharper focus and there will be hope and real prospects for achieving personal goals.

An inclusive organisation will actively manage risk from a human rights perspective. There will be a recognition that living in inadequate housing on a depressing estate with no job, friends or leisure pursuits is a high-risk lifestyle.

The inclusive mental health service will create real opportunities for people with mental health problems to access a decent quality of life, and will develop partnerships with housing providers, employers, college staff and civic organisations. The boundaries of confidentiality and disclosure will be explored through a carefully negotiated process that empowers service users.

Work colleagues, acquaintances and friends will then exchange personal support to the service user and they will contribute some degree of monitoring and give early warning of the person's deterioration. This is not a matter of recruiting neighbours to a '1984 style' thought police, but rather the informal encouragement which many of us enjoy from time to time when a colleague or a friend urges us to visit the doctor about that persistent cough (MacDonald–Wilson and Whitman, 1995).

Discharge mechanisms and eligibility criteria will be stringently checked to ensure that people are not disqualified from receiving a service that they need, or encouraged to remain within services for fear of subsequent disqualification. Individualised services that build on service users' aspirations for recovery will gradually increase service capacity as more people emerge from a long-term relationship with services into a valued lifestyle in the community.

Performance management

We have already referred to the need for empowerment of direct care staff in the organisation, and this naturally suggests flattened hierarchies, devolved decision making and some degree of self-management within teams. However, these trends have sometimes been used as a Trojan horse for the imposition of heavy workloads and a victim-blaming culture.

An inclusive organisation will care for the needs of all the staff by making best use of their time and skills as part of the adoption of a balanced lifestyle. Incidentally, we have anecdotal evidence to suggest that many people who become involved in inclusive and person-centred practice often apply the same principles to their own lives and take courageous and creative decisions about their lifestyle and career. This means that some staff leave the organisation to pursue their ambitions while others decline both promotion opportunities and overtime.

 © THE SAINSBURY CENTRE FOR MENTAL HEALTH, 2002

While many organisations currently pay lip service to social inclusion, the essential tasks are not often found on job descriptions, and activity-monitoring systems rarely report on the transition of service users into valued roles in the community.

In an inclusive organisation job descriptions and activity monitoring systems for direct care staff include the components of inclusion work, such as community mapping, capacity building and support work with individuals who are seeking to increase their participation in the life of the community.

This is a critical component in an increasingly evidence-based service framework. In addition, workload and performance management information will be shared with users and partner organisations, and users will have ready access to their files (Department of Health, 2000a) and be able to update planning documentation.

Instead of the line management task being used as an observation platform for the detection of poor quality work, the focus is upon individual workers consulting their senior colleagues in order to maintain professionalism and their high personal standards of practice.

Information from staff, including appraisals, exit interviews and consultation exercises is systematically analysed and acted upon. Innovation will be encouraged and rewarded in an atmosphere where mistakes are treated as learning opportunities.

Policies keep people safe, but promote the unique cultural identity, sexuality, interests, abilities and talents of each person served by the organisation. Policies also promote sensible risk-taking, rather than limiting opportunities for imaginative problem solving by staff. An inclusive organisation welcomes service evaluation and contributions from service users, advocates and the friends, relatives and social contacts of service users.

Within an inclusive organisation, first-line managers will have strong links with community organisations and use them frequently to support service user engagement with others who share their chosen identity in the community. Year by year the network of contacts with community partners will grow and contact with the mental health service will be initiated by the community agencies as they increasingly value the contribution made by service users.

Resource management

The new flexibilities arising from the *Health Act 1999* will be fully exploited within an inclusive mental health service. Whereas at one time pooled budgets were unusual and some finance departments had little experience of them, an inclusive organisation will have achieved pooling with probity. This will mean that where any service fails to meet the required standards, then remedial action is quickly taken or the service is transferred to a new provider.

Perhaps more importantly, pooled budgets, joint funded projects and partnership agreements will have been extended to create close working links with other sectors such as education, employment, housing and leisure providers. The result will be seamless support for people to enable movement from intensive mental health support to a positive and full life in the community.

The budget profile will show that the organisation is investing in inclusion. This will be manifest as a significant spend on inclusive projects and services as well as investment in relevant clinical audit, research, library materials and service innovations.

There will be a distinct effort to recruit staff that hold inclusive personal values and practice in a creative manner. The training programme will further develop inclusive strategies and creativity within individuals and teams. Service users will be employed in the labour force, and will participate as both trainers and trainees in staff development events.

Over time, the organisation will make increasing accommodations to enable the employment of people with mental health problems (Department of Health, 2000b). While staff and service users are protected from undue intrusion into their personal lives, the spectrum of relationship from staff member, through volunteer to friend will be redefined to clarify the way in which staff may engage with service users in an unpaid capacity.

As the mental health agency journeys towards a more inclusive approach, individual work with service users is increasingly favoured. Fewer resources are invested in congregate services and arrangements which place people far from their natural community, and these are rigorously and frequently reviewed in order to bring people back home whenever possible.

The range of individual choice grows ever wider. Contact with community agencies bears fruit as they also make increasing accommodations to respond to the needs of mental health service users who are engaged in their activities.

Closer relationships lead to a reduction in stigma and improvements in attitude so that community organisations begin to invest in joint projects that offer inclusive opportunities to people with mental health problems. As a result, additional resources are levered in. Service users become a stronger resource in support of the move towards inclusion as they increasingly recommend opportunities to their peers and provide support to one another in taking up positive roles.

 © THE SAINSBURY CENTRE FOR MENTAL HEALTH, 2002

Strategic management

The fundamental attitudes of senior management within the organisation will subtly control the direction and speed of change. Within an inclusive organisation the top management will hold a personal conviction of the importance of inclusion, and will promote these beliefs. In addition to occasional visits to service areas, they will have sustained contact with the actual experiences and lifestyles of some service users in order to keep in touch with what is important.

Senior management will work for organisational coherence – to ensure that inclusion is supported throughout all levels and sections of the agency – and to ensure that it harmonises with other goals. They will be alert to inconsistencies and counter-productive elements of their system and will be eager to identify and discontinue any practices that inhibit care improvements. Rewards will go to innovative, creative people who promote inclusion.

Decision making within the organisation is a shared process. The experience and viewpoint of service users, direct care staff and other stakeholders is increasingly valued in project design, training and marketing events. Year on year the organisation reaches more effectively towards people who are traditionally hard to engage and offers more diverse opportunities. For users with needs that are hard to meet, service specifications and financial incentives are improved to encourage the service to be provided.

Big and inclusive

It has been suggested that big bureaucracies like social services departments or NHS bodies are toxic environments for inclusive practice. Proponents of this view argue that the bureaucracy can only support the inclusion agenda by providing funds to small, independent bodies for them to do the work. This position seems weak for the following reasons:

- The funding agency will continue to require a good understanding of inclusion in order to select appropriate indicators for monitoring the sub-contracted work.
- It is unlikely that the large bureaucracies will devolve a significant proportion of their work, and so inclusive projects will remain marginal.
- Small, independent sector bodies may be no more innovative than large agencies. Indeed, they may expend so much energy on survival that few resources are left for innovation.
- As innovative organisations age, they are at serious risk of becoming encrusted with restrictive policies and limited to preserving their original idea.

© THE SAINSBURY CENTRE FOR MENTAL HEALTH, 2002

These arguments persuade us that we need to continue the process of defining the characteristics of an inclusive organisation, rather than assuming that 'inclusive' is synonymous with 'small', 'independent' or 'young'.

The description of an inclusive organisation may seem laughably beyond reach. However, it is our contention that much conflict within organisations occurs due to the lack of a shared goal. By offering this dream of an inclusive organisation we hope to show how many of the current policy imperatives and pressures upon mental health services can be drawn together within a coherent paradigm. We offer this as a compelling image.

Criteria for an inclusive organisation

Any large organisation or inter-agency partnership can be rated on a scale between exclusive and inclusive. The scale overleaf contrasts a well-functioning and successful organisation that has not yet adopted an inclusive approach with one that has taken on the full ramifications of an inclusive philosophy. The 'exclusive' organisation pictured on the left-hand column is successful on many counts, but it is not promoting inclusion. You may wish to use the scale with a diverse group. Privately rate your own agency and then discuss your scores. The discussion may be more important than the scores!

 © THE SAINSBURY CENTRE FOR MENTAL HEALTH, 2002

Criteria for an inclusive organisation

	Successful but excluding organisations tend to		Including organisations tend to
A	Reach some sections of the community with information, opportunities, goods, services, and employment.	**Comprehensive** 1–2 3–4	Serve the whole community. Service users are employed in the service, sit on management teams and monitor quality. Information and opportunity to influence the organisation is freely available.
B	Focus on the provision of health and social care.	**Holistic** 1–2 3–4	Work towards everyone having the chance to enjoy good health, develop skills, earn a wage and live in safety.
C	Promote support between people who use services.	**Roles** 1–2 3–4	Promote the maintenance and further development of positive roles in the community and relationships between people who use services and other citizens.
D	Focus on assessment of needs, eligibility criteria and review of interventions. Most people receive standard package of services in segregated settings.	**Unique** 1–2 3–4	Attend to people's life ambitions in partnership with informal supporters. Most people get a unique package of support to maintain their life in the mainstream community.
E	Getting help often means a disruption to personal routines and relationships.	**Service** 1–2 3–4	Support is offered in a manner which nurtures personal roles and relationships beyond the service system.
F	Staff job descriptions and monitoring systems track the delivery of health and social care processes and outcome.	**Monitoring** 1–2 3–4	Job descriptions and performance indicators track inclusive outcomes for service users – a job, friends, a decent home, personal life targets.
G	Thorough supervision systems identify staff limitations and repair with appropriate training.	**Creative** 1–2 3–4	Staff are supported through balanced lifestyles, mentoring and encouragement to solve problems using imagination and creativity.
H	Pooled budgets, joint funded projects and partnership work are rare and only with similar agencies.	**Partnership** 1–2 3–4	Support diverse community organisations that assist people to engage with them and move freely from intensive mental health support into a full life in the community.

 © THE SAINSBURY CENTRE FOR MENTAL HEALTH, 2002

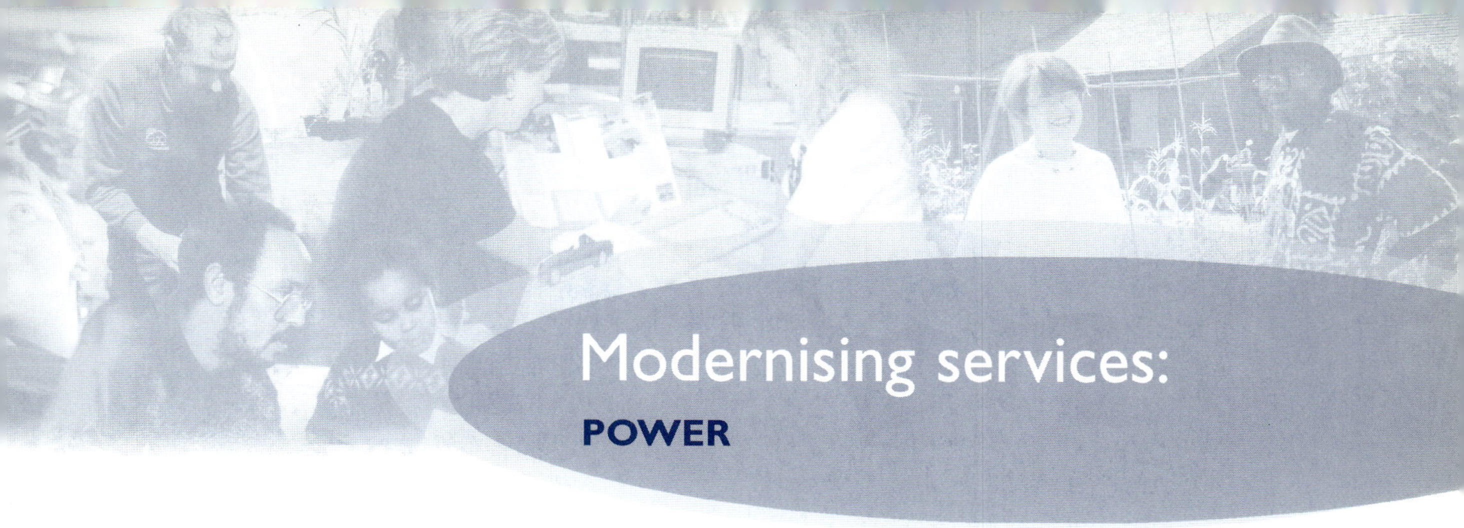

Modernising services:
POWER

Ron Coleman

"To include or not include, is the question – or why bother, as they will only screw up anyway?"

I view the concept of inclusion within a wider context than mental health. As the chief executive officer of an independent organisation that has a mission statement promoting an inclusive society, I must confess to feeling fearful that we are embarking once again down the road of buzzword led policy. The recent history of empowerment as a construct in mental health provides a good starting point to begin a debate on inclusion and the impact that the notion of inclusion can have on mental health services.

The empowerment lobby had a very sound case for the approach they adopted on the issue of 'empowering users'. It was based on the clear precept that users were powerless, needed to gain more power and autonomy, which would in turn increase the choice that users could make about the services that they received. It is clear to me that those that promoted the ideas of empowerment did so for all of the right reasons.

Taken, not given

The first hurdle we face in an inclusion process then is finding a way to take back power. There is an ongoing attempt to address this power issue within mental health. However, since this well-intentioned start, empowerment in general and empowering users in particular has become the political correctness of the mental health system. While the language has changed, this political correctness has not led to a change in practice or delivered autonomy to the service user.

One of the reasons for the failure of this 'empowering approach' is rooted in our failure to understand one of the fundamental truths about power: power is taken, not given. If we look at the history of many of the campaigns for freedom or equality we can see that it was the perceived threat to the establishment (those who wield power) that made the establishment cede power.

 © THE SAINSBURY CENTRE FOR MENTAL HEALTH, 2002

Women in the United Kingdom are a case in point: they won the vote – they were not given the vote. The role of the suffragettes in this fight for emancipation cannot be denied (though the establishment try to do so). Women were jailed, forcibly fed and died in the battle to win the vote. It was their sacrifice that forced the state to concede the vote.

Similarly, gay people had to fight to win the right to live a particular lifestyle, and so they demanded and took the right to live their lives as they saw fit. They did this by 'coming out of the closet' and demanding acceptance. This was carried out against a background in which homosexuality was deemed to be a mental illness until the early 1970s. It was the sheer volume of those coming out that forced the law to be changed.

The twentieth century also saw many colonies claiming independence from their colonial masters. Many of these had to fight bloody wars to achieve their independence. It was not so much that these colonies were given freedom but rather that they took their freedom and the colonisers merely gave way to the inevitable.

The same principles can be applied to the issues of power faced by those who use mental health services leading to the conclusion that the reclamation of power is something that is essential in any inclusion process. Taking or reclaiming power does not have to conflict with the 'empower' approach that has been adopted by the system and the two approaches can work together. These issues can be explored using dialectical methodology.

The ideas surrounding the need to empower users are based on an admission by professionals that power is an issue. The real problem is not in their understanding that power is an issue but in the fact that they see the service user at its core.

It is here that their analysis is flawed, for it is not the professionals' role to give power to clients. Their role should be to give up the power they hold over service users and by doing so create the conditions in which service users can reclaim power for themselves. Likewise it is not the role of the service user to passively wait to be empowered but to be active in taking back their personal power. This is not and will never be an easy thing for professionals or service users to do.

Defensive practice

The problem that users and professionals face when dealing with the issues of giving up power should not be underestimated. Due to the way mental health systems are organised professionals are forced to work within a system that is based on defensive practice.

 © THE SAINSBURY CENTRE FOR MENTAL HEALTH, 2002

Defensive practice by its very nature does not encourage any form of risk taking and indeed it does the opposite and ensures that practice is conservative at best and oppressive at its worst. The 'no risk' strategy creates the 'no recovery' culture and leads to the very power struggle that all sides claim they wish to end.

'Take no risks' has become the new dogma of mental health services, and as long as this is the case inclusion will not be a realistic option for many.

As a service user throughout the 1980s and into the 1990s, I was part of the great empowerment experimental experience, and if I were now asked to reflect on how that impacted on the care and treatment that I received, I would have to say not at all. For all the talk of choice, my psychiatrist still had the power to block my desire for talking treatment because he did not think that it would benefit me. I believe that it is therefore correct to conclude that the concept of empowerment was just that – a concept, not a reality.

There is a similar challenge facing us in the inclusion debate and that is whether we can really gift people inclusion. Or can inclusion be based within a single issue such as health, gender, race or poverty? Will inclusion become bogged down in the mire that equal opportunities found itself in the 1980s, where it was seen as the responsibility of an individual or group rather than the responsibility of all within society? Is there a danger then that inclusion (like empowerment or recovery) will be seen as an event or a movement rather than a process?

An inclusive workplace

Much of the debate within my own organisation is around these types of questions. We have not found the answers but we have learned that we need to clarify what inclusion means to us as an organisation.

One thing we have agreed is that inclusion is not the problem – the problem is exclusion. In the context of my organisation I have concluded that I was guilty of excluding individuals within my company both in the decision making process and by the disparity in pay within the workforce. Through re-organisation we have attempted to deal with both issues.

We now have in place a process of planning company development that involves everyone. We also concluded that the minimum wage was not a decent living wage and introduced the European Decency Threshold as our minimum wage for everyone. At the time of writing this currently stands at £7·40 an hour or around £14,500 a year.

The fact that the bulk of our workforce has or has had mental health problems was not the driving force for these decisions, rather it was our desire to have real fairness in the workplace. We are mindful of everyone's well-being within the company and this means all of the staff and not just those who are 'out' about their mental health problems. For example, we have two extra days holiday a year that we call duvet days – a time when an employee can simply stay under the duvet, rather than coming into work. These days are available to every member of the organisation and are about maintaining the mental well-being of the entire workforce – not just about looking after those with a diagnosis.

The danger of trying to make mental health a special case is that by default we create structures that exclude and become part of the problem rather than part of the solution. People with mental distress may be in the community, but still directed, supervised and controlled by powerful professionals.

Can mental health services be inclusive when the drive within legislation is towards a more coercive and alienating system? This is a question that must be answered if we are to be wary of trying to dress up exclusion in inclusive clothing. In proposed legislation there is much talk of the system being governed by the best interest of the client. This sounds laudable, a person-centred approach to mental health at long last, but the sting is in the tail as it will be the doctor who will determine best interest. Power has not moved, so inclusive efforts will fail.

We need now more than ever to strive for an inclusive society and this must begin within each of us. There is no point in continuing this debate until first we acknowledge the issue of power within mental health services. Secondly, we must be prepared to be honest about the vested interest in maintaining that power balance within the system and finally we must give up our own vested interest in maintaining the status quo. Then and only then can inclusion become a reality – not just within mental health, but also within society.

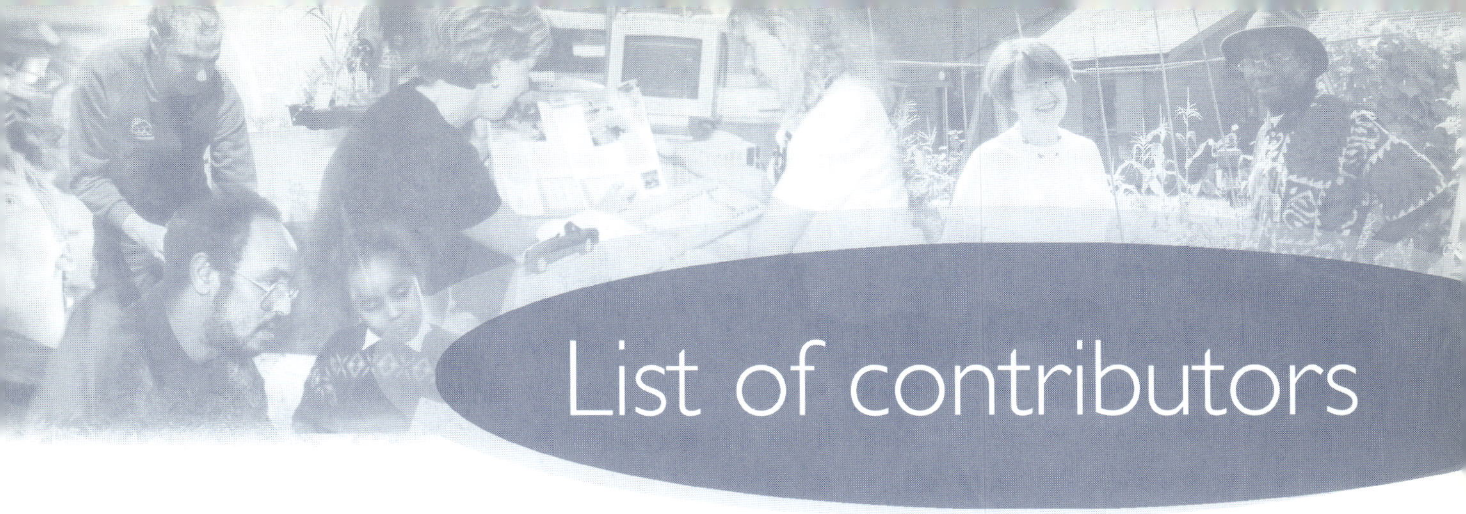

List of contributors

Anna Barnes
Project Manager
East Sussex County Healthcare NHS Trust
St Ann's Centre, 729 The Ridge
St Leonard's on Sea, Sussex TN37 7RD

Peter Bates
National Development Team, Albion Wharf
Albion Street, Manchester M1 5LN
Tel: 0161 228 7055
email: pbates@ndt.org.uk

The NDT works with learning disability and mental health services and users to provide training and consultancy on empowerment, social inclusion and quality lifestyles.

Roy Batten, Service User, Bromley Mind

David Boyle
Associate, New Economics Foundation
Cinnamon House, 6–8 Cole Street
London SE1 4YH
email: david.boyle@neweconomics.org

Dr Jan Burns
Centre for Applied Social
& Psychological Development
Canterbury Christ Church University
College, Salomons, Broomhill Road
Southborough, Tunbridge Wells
Kent TN3 0TG

Pam Buttrey
Head Occupational Therapist
Oxleas NHS Trust

Ron Coleman
Managing Director, Keepwell Ltd
City Works, Alfred Street
Gloucester GL1 4DF
Tel: 01452 551147
www.keepwell-uk.com

Jon Cribbens
House Manager, Community Options
email: Com.optionsts@pop3.poptel.org.uk

Dr Fabian A. Davis
Consultant Clinical Psychologist
Department of Clinical Psychology
Bromley Mental Health Services
Oxleas NHS Trust, 38 Mason's Hill
Bromley, Kent BR2 9JG
email: 100255.3512@compuserve.com

Alison Faulkner
Head of Service User Initiatives
The Mental Health Foundation,
20–21 Cornwall Terrace
London NW1 4QL

Michael Fletcher
Bromley Advocacy Project
email: www.bap@advoproject.fsnet.co.uk

Dr Lynne Friedli
Chief Executive, **mentality**
134–138 Borough High Street
London SE1 1LB
Tel: 020 7716 6777
www.mentality.org.uk
mentality is the first national charity dedicated to promoting mental health.

Elizabeth Gale
Policy and Development Manager
mentality

Andrew Gibb
Bridge-builder, *Mainstream*
Imagine, 25 Hope Street
Liverpool L1 9BQ
Tel: 0151 709 8643

K. Gilyead
Pentreath Industries Ltd
20 Higher Bugle, Bugle
St Austell PL26 8PY
Tel: 01726 850565
email: pentreath@pentreath.co.uk

Maurice Harker
Housing and Support Partnership
78a High Street, Witney OX28 6HL
Tel: 01993 705012
email: harker@housingandsupport.co.uk

Sarah Hean
Florence Nightingale School of Nursing and Midwifery, King's College London
James Clarke Maxwell Building
57 Waterloo Road, London SE1 8WA
email: sarah.hean@kcl.ac.uk

Jacqueline Henderson
Executive Director, Learning and Skills Council, London Central, Centrepoint
103 New Oxford Street
London WC1A 1DR

Louise Holden
PALS Officer and Service User
Oxleas NHS Trust

Jon Hyslop
Manager, Oxfordshire Mental Health Matters
OMHM provides information, advocacy and low-cost training on mental health issues to the county of Oxfordshire.
Enquiries: 01865 728981
email: omhm@oxford-mentalhealth.org

Ann Jackson
Senior Practice Development Fellow
RCN Institute Mental Health Programme
c/o Radcliffe Infirmary, Woodstock Road
Oxford OX2 6HE
email: ann.jackson@rcn.org.uk

Kathryn James
Development Officer, Learning and Health
NIACE, 21 De Montfort Street
Leicester LE1 7GE
Tel: 0116 2044281
email: kathryn.james@niace.org.uk

Phil Jones
Clubhouse Member and Service User
Horizon House, Bromley

Ken Jue
Chief Executive Officer
Monadnock Family Services
64 Main Street, Keene
New Hampshire 03431, USA
Tel: 603 357 6878
Fax: 603 357 6896, email: kjue@mfs.org

Iain Kitchener
Deputy House Manager
Community Options

 © THE SAINSBURY CENTRE FOR MENTAL HEALTH, 2002

Louise Knox
Development Officer
Pentreath Industries Ltd
20 Higher Bugle, Bugle, St Austell PL26 8PY
Tel: 01726 850565
email: pentreath@pentreath.co.uk

Peter Lindley
Deputy Director of Practice Development and Training
The Sainsbury Centre for Mental Health
134–138 Borough High Street
London SE1 1LB

Ruth Marriott
Health Services Manager
Youth Enquiry Service, 14–16 Union Street
Derry's Cross, Plymouth PL1 2SR
Tel: 01752 206626
email: marriottruth@hotmail.com

Dr Allyson McCollam
Director of Research
Scottish Development Centre for Mental Health
17A Graham St, Edinburgh EH6 5QN
Tel: 0131 555 5959
email: allyson@sdcmh.org.uk

Helen Macklin
Clubhouse Worker
email: horizonclubhouse@bun.com

Clive Miller
Senior Fellow in Organisational Development, Office for Public Management, 252b Gray's Inn Road
London WC1X 8XG
Tel: 020 7239 7915
email: cmiller@opm.co.uk

Kim Minter, Sector Liaison Worker
Bromley User Group

David Morris
Head of Citizenship and Community Programme
The Sainsbury Centre for Mental Health
134–138 Borough High Street
London SE1 1LB

Kevin Pace
Community Mental Health Nurse
Oxleas NHS Trust

Karen Pavey
Service User Researcher, Oxleas NHS Trust

Rachel Perkins
Clinical Director of General Adult Services and Consultant Clinical Psychologist
South West London and St George's Mental Health NHS Trust

Vanessa Pinfold
Health Services Research Department
Institute of Psychiatry, Denmark Hill
London SE5 8AF

Peter Rainford
Metamorphosis Change Management Consultancy
email: peterj.rainford@btopenworld.com

Zoe Reed
Executive Director, Developing Organisation and Community
South London and Maudsley NHS Trust
Tel: 020 7919 2435
email: Zoe.Reed@slam-tr.nhs.uk

Julie Repper
Senior Research Fellow/Lead Research Nurse, University of Sheffield/Community Health Sheffield, School of Health and Related Research, Regent Court
Regent Street, Sheffield S1 4DA

 © THE SAINSBURY CENTRE FOR MENTAL HEALTH, 2002

Pete Ritchie
Scottish Human Services Trust
1a Washington Court
Edinburgh EH11 2HA
Tel: 0131 538 7717
email: pritchie@shstrust.org.uk
www.shstrust.org.uk.

Penny Robertson
Chief Executive, Pentreath Industries Ltd
20 Higher Bugle, Bugle, St Austell
Cornwall PL26 8PY
Tel: 01726 850565
email: penny@pentreath.co.uk

Liz Sayce
Director of Policy and Research
Disability Rights Commission
222 Gray's Inn Road, London WC1X 8HL

Dr Justine Schneider
Senior Lecturer, Centre for
Applied Social Studies
University of Durham
Durham DH1 3HL
email: justine.schneider@durham.ac.uk

Fran Silvestri
Former Chief Executive Officer
Monadnock Family Service, USA.
Does project work with Monadnock
and is a senior consultant with the Centre
of Community Change International.
Contact at 1/54 Millen Ave
Pakuranga, New Zealand
Tel: 09 527 3966
Fax: 09 527 4433.
Mobile: 025 782279
email: fran@pl.net

Nikki Slater
Day Service Worker, Bromley Mind

Richard K. Sutton
Formerly of Survivors Speak Out, London,
and Independent User Consultant

Paul Taylor
The Red House Partnership
Rushbed Cottage, Crawshawbooth
Rossendale, Lancs BB4 8LX
email: paul@rushbed.co.uk
The Red House Partnership is engaged
in community capacity building.

Sara Weech
Commissioning Manager for Mental Health
Isle of Wight PCG, Whitecroft
Sandy Lane, Newport
Isle of Wight PO30 3ED

Julia White
Associate Consultant, Scottish
Development Centre for Mental Health
17A Graham Street, Edinburgh EH6 5QN
Tel: 0131 555 5959

Toni Wilkinson
Chief Executive, Hastings and
St Leonard's Primary Care Group
PO Box 124, St Leonard's on Sea
Sussex TN38 0XZ

Melba Wilson
Policy Director
Mind, 15–19 Broadway
London E15 4BQ
Tel: 020 8215 2264
email: m.wilson@mind.org.uk

 © THE SAINSBURY CENTRE FOR MENTAL HEALTH, 2002

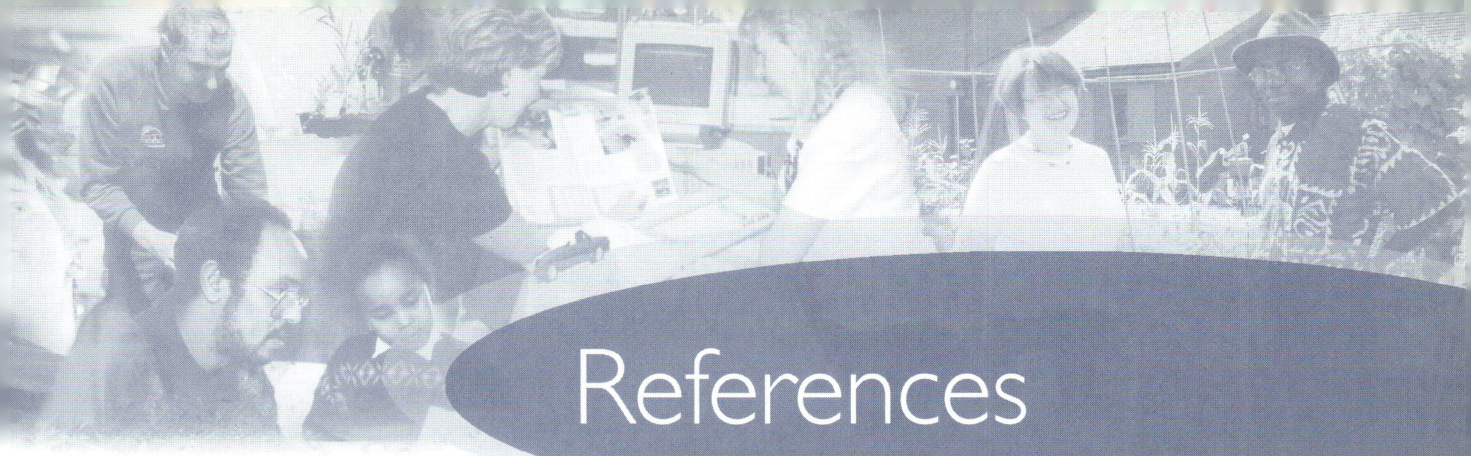

References

Ager, A. (1990) *The Life Experiences Checklist Manual.* Windsor: NFER–Nelson.

Amado, A. N. (ed.) (1993) *Friendships and Community Connections Between People with and without Developmental Disabilities.* Baltimore: Paul H Brookes.

Anderson, I., Sim, D. (2000) Housing and Social Exclusion: the changing debate. In *Social Exclusion and Housing: Context and Challenges,* 6–21. Coventry: Chartered Institute of Housing and Housing Studies Association.

Anderson, J., Dayson, D., Wills, W., Gooch, C., Margolius, O., O'Driscoll, C., Leff, J. (1993). The TAPS project. 13: clinical and social outcomes of long-stay psychiatric patients after one year in the community. *British Journal of Psychiatry,* **162** (supplement 19), 45–56.

Angermeyer, M. C. (2001) Paper to *Together Against Stigma* Conference. Leipzig: 2001.

Angermeyer, M.C., Matschinger, H. (1996) The effect of personal experience with mental illness on the attitude towards individuals suffering from mental disorders. *Social Psychiatry and Psychiatric Epidemiology,* **31** 321–326.

Arboleda–Florez (2001) Paper to *Together Against Stigma* Conference. Leipzig: 2001.

Audit Commission (1998) *Messages for Managers: learning the lessons from Joint Reviews of Social Services.* London: Audit Commission.

Audit Commission (1999) *Making Connections: learning the lessons from Joint Reviews of Social Services.* London: Social Services Inspectorate, Audit Commission, Department of Health and National Assembly for Wales.

Barkham, P. (2000) Disability Benefits. *Guardian Unlimited* (April 20).

Barnes, C., Mercer, G. (1997) *Doing Disability Research.* Leeds: The Disability Press.

Bates, P. (2000) Introducing Circles of Friends. *A Life in the Day,* **4** (4) 20–22.

Bates, P., Repper, J. (2001) Social inclusion – a framework for evaluation. *A Life in the Day,* **5** (2) 18–23.

Bates P. (2002, forthcoming) *A Real Asset.* Manchester: National Development Team.

Battram, A., (1997) *Navigating Complexity.* London: Industrial Society.

Becker, D.R. Drake, R.E. (1993). *The individual placement and support model of supported employment.* Dartford: New Hampshire.

Beresford, P., Wallcraft, J. (1997). Psychiatric System Survivors and Emancipatory Research: issues, overlaps and differences. In Barnes, C., Mercer, G. *Doing Disability Research.* Leeds: The Disability Press.

Beyer, S., Goodere, L., Kilsby, M. (1996) *Costs & Benefits of Supported Employment Agencies: Findings from a national survey.* Employment Service Research Series R37. London: Stationery Office.

 © THE SAINSBURY CENTRE FOR MENTAL HEALTH, 2002

Bond, G.R.(1998) Principles of the individual placement and support model: empirical support. *Psychiatric Rehabilitation Journal*, **22** (1) 11–23.

Bond, G.R., Drake, R.E., Meuser, K.T., Becker, D.R. (1997) An update on supported employment for people with severe mental illness. *Psychiatric Services*, **48** 333–346.

Bond, S., Davis, F.A. (1997) *The Community Rehabilitation Service: what do users think of it and Ideal Rehabilitation Services?* Oxleas NHS Trust.

Braisby, D., Echlin, R., Hill, S., Smith, H. (1988) *Changing Futures. Housing and Support Services for People Discharged from Psychiatric Hospitals.* London: King Edward's Hospital Fund.

Brost, M., Johnson, T., Wagner, L., Deprey, R. (1982) *Getting to Know You – One Approach to Service Assessment and Planning for Individuals with Disabilities.* Madison: Wisconsin Coalition for Advocacy.

Brown, G.W., Harris T. (1978) *Social Origins of Depression.* London: Tavistock.

Buchanon, J. (1995) Social Support and Schizophrenia: A review of the Literature. *Archives of Psychiatric Nursing.* **ix** (2) (April) 1995 68–76.

Bullen and Onyx (1998) *Measuring Social Capital in Five Communities in NSW – A Practitioner's Guide.* http://www.mapl.com.au/A13.htm.

Bunch, G. (1997) *Inclusion: Recent Research.* Toronto: Inclusion Press.

Burt, R. S. (1997) The Contingent Value of Social Capital. *Administrative Science Quarterly,* **42** 339–365.

Byrne, P. (2000) Stigma of mental illness and ways of diminishing it. *Advances in Psychiatric Treatment,* **6** 65–72.

Cabinet Office (1998) *Bringing Britain Together: a national strategy for neighbourhood renewal.* Cm 4045 September 1998. London: Cabinet Office.

Cabinet Office (2000) *National Strategy for Neighbourhood Renewal: a framework for consultation.* Report by the Social Exclusion Unit. London: Cabinet Office.

Campbell, P. (2000) The role of users of psychiatric services in service development – influence not power. *Psychiatric Bulletin*, **25** 87–88.

Canadian Council on Social Development. Assessing the effectiveness of deinstitutionalization: substantive and methodological conclusions from the research literature. *Deinstitutionalization: Costs and effects*, 75–102. Ottawa: Canadian Council on Social Development.

Carling, P.J. (1995) *Return to Community*. New York: The Guilford Press.

Carpenter, J., Sbaraini, S. (1997) *Choice, information and dignity: Involving users and carers in care management in mental health.* Bristol: Policy Press.

Carson, J., Dowling, F., Glynn, T., Oliver, N. (1994) The role of normalisation in psychiatric rehabilitation: an empirical investigation. *Care in Place*, **1** (3) 231–243.

Coleman, J. S. (1988) Social Capital in the Creation of Human Capital. *American Journal of Sociology*, **94** S95–S120.

Collier, P. (1998) *Social Capital and Poverty.* http://www.worldbank.org/poverty/scapital/.

Cooper, H., Arber, S., Fee, L., Ginn, J. (1999) *Social Capital for Health – The influence of social support and social capital on health – A review and analysis of British data.* London: Health Education Authority.

Cournos, F. (1987) The impact of environmental factors on outcome in residential settings. *Hospital and Community Psychiatry*, **38** (8) 848–852.

Cowley, S., Billings, J., Forbes, A., Griffiths, P., Hean, S., Maben, J., Murrells, T. (2000) *An examination of the potential to identify an instrument reflecting measurable attributes of social capital.* Research in progress. London: King's College.

Crisp, A., Gelder, M., Rix, S. *et al.*, (2000) Stigmatisation of people with mental illness. *British Journal of Psychiatry,* **177** 4–7.

Crowther, R., Marshall, M., Bond, G., Huxley, P. (2000) *Vocational rehabilitation for people with severe mental disorders.* Cochrane Review, Cochrane Library.

Cullen, D., Carson, J., Holloway, F., Towey, A., Jumbo, A., Smellie, N., Glynn, T. (1977) Community and hospital residential care: a comparative evaluation. *Irish Journal of Psychological Medicine,* **14** (3) 92–98.

Dansereau, J., Duteau, E., Ely, P., Flynn, R. J. (1990) Evaluation des programmes residentiels en sante mentale dans l'Outaouais. Hull, Quebec: Conseil regional de la sante et des services sociaux de l'Outaouais. In Flynn, R.J. (ed). (1994), Chapter 14. A comprehensive review of research with PASS and PASSING. *The Ottowa Conference: 25 Years of Normalisation.* Available from: RFLYNN@locutus.cc.uottowa.ca.

Davis, F.A. (1999) Measuring need according to the 5 service accomplishments: The properties and utility of the Support Needs Questionnaire. In *A Course of Readings for Professional and Graduate Education in Effective Community Care for People with Mental Health Problems. Appendix to Volume 2: Assessment Schedules and Related Material.* London: The Sainsbury Centre for Mental Health.

Davis, F.A. (2001) Revalorisation: What experiences, resources and supports contribute to successful social reinclusion and a return to valued social status for people with severe and enduring mental illness. *Proceedings of the British Psychological Society,* **9** (2) 134.

Davis, F.A., Burns, J., Lindley, P., Sutton, R.K. (In press). Need According to the 5 Accomplishments. The Properties and Utility of the Support Needs Questionnaire (SNQ).

Davis, F.A., Lindley, P. (1991) *Individual Service Review: planning and quality assurance.* Paper presented at a National Conference on Quality Assurance. Nursing and Quality Assurance Directorate. London: SETRHA.

Deegan, P. (1996) Recovery as a Journey of the Heart. *Psychiatric Rehabilitation Journal,* **19** (3) 91–97.

Department of the Environment and Department of Health (1997) *Housing and Community Care; establishing a strategic framework.* London: Department of the Environment, Department of Health.

Department of Health (1988) *Caring for People: Community Care in the Next Decade and Beyond.* London: HMSO.

Department of Health (1989) *Working for Patients.* London: HMSO.

Department of Health (1990) *The Care Programme Approach for People with a Mental Illness,* HC (90) 24/LASSL 90 (11) London: Department of Health.

Department of Health (1998a) *Modernising Social Services – promoting independence, improving practice, raising standards.* London: HSMO

Department of Health (1998b) *Modernising Mental Health Services: Safe, Sound and Supportive.* London: HMSO.

Department of Health (1999a) *Modernising the Care Programme Approach.* London: Department of Health.

Department of Health (1999b) *National Service Framework for Mental Health: modern standards and service models.* London: HMSO.

Department of Health (2000) *The NHS Plan: a plan for investment, a plan for reform.* London: HMSO.

 © THE SAINSBURY CENTRE FOR MENTAL HEALTH, 2002

Department of Health (March 2000a) *Data Protection Act 1998: Guidance to Social Services.* London: Department of Health.

Department of Health (2000b) *Looking beyond labels: Widening the employment opportunities for disabled people in the new NHS.* London: Department of Health.

Department of Health (2001a) *Safety First: Five Year Report of the National Confidential Inquiry and Homicide by People with Mental Illness.* London: Department of Health.

Department of Health (2001b) *Making it happen: a guide to delivering mental health promotion.* London: Department of Health.

Department of Health and Home Office (2000) *Reforming the Mental Health Act.* London: HMSO.

Department of Work and Pensions (2001) *Recruiting Benefit Claimaints: Qualitative Research with Employers in ONE Pilot Area.* Research Series Paper No 150, prepared by Bunt, K., Shury, J., Vivian, D. London: Department of Work and Pensions.

Dodd & Loeb (1998) In Naidoo, J., & Wills, J. *Practicing Health Promotion: Dilemmas and Challenges.* London: Ballière Tindel.

Dodd, J., Sandell, R. (2001) *Including Museums: perspectives on museums, galleries and social inclusion.* Leicester: Research Centre for Museums and Galleries, University of Leicester.

Drake, R. E., McHugo, G., Bebout, R., Becker, D., Harris, M., Bond, G., Quimby, E. (1999a) A randomised clinical trial of supported employment for inner-city patients with severe mental disorders. *Archives of General Psychiatry*, **56** 627–633.

Drake, R.E., Becker, D.R., Clark, R.E., Mueser, K.T. (1999b) Research on the Individual Placement and Support model of Supported Employment. *Psychiatric Quarterly*, **70** 289–301.

Drury, V. (2000) Cognitive Behaviour Therapy in Early Psychosis. In Birchwood, M., Fowler, D., Jackson, G. (eds). *Early Intervention in Psychosis,* 188. Chichester: Wiley.

Dunn, S. (1999) *Creating accepting communities: report of the MIND enquiry into social exclusion and mental health problems.* London: Mind publications.

Ellison, M., Pierson, C. (1998) *Developments in British Social Policy.* London: Macmillan.

Fadden, G. (1997) Implementation of family interventions in routine clinical practice following staff training programmes: A major cause for concern. *Journal of Mental Health*, **6** 599–612.

Faulkner, A. (1997) *Knowing our own Minds.* London: Mental Health Foundation.

Faulkner, A., Layzell, S. (2000) *Strategies for living: report of user led research into people's strategies for living with mental distress.* London: Mental Health Foundation.

Felce, D. (1988) Evaluating the Extent of Community Integration Following the Provision of Staffed Residential Alternatives to Institutional Care. *Irish Journal of Pathology*, **9** (2) 346–360.

Forrest, R., Kearns, A. (1999) *Joined-up Places? Social cohesion and neighbourhood regeneration.* York: Joseph Rowntree Foundation.

Foucault, M. (1965) *Madness and Civilisation.* New York: Random House.

Friedli, L. (2000) Mental health promotion: re-thinking the evidence base. *The Mental Health Review,* **5** (3) 15–18.

Golden, S.J. (1982). *Normalisation in mental health community residences.* Unpublished doctoral dissertation. University of Rhode Island.

 © THE SAINSBURY CENTRE FOR MENTAL HEALTH, 2002

Gordon, D., Levitas, R., Pantazis, C., Payne, S., Townsend, P., Bradshaw, J., Middleton, S., Bramley, G., Bridgwood, A., Maher, J., Rowlands, O. (1999); *Poverty and Social Exclusion Survey for Britain.* http://qb.soc.surrey.ac.uk/surveys/pse/pseintro.htm.

Gowman, N. (1999) *Healthy Neighbourhoods.* London: King's Fund.

Granovetter, M. S. (1973) The Strength of Weak Ties. *American Journal of Sociology*, **78** 1360–1380.

Grant, T. (ed.) (2000) *Physical activity and mental health: national consensus statements and guidelines for practice.* London: Somerset Health Authority/Health Education Authority.

Griffiths, R. (1988) *Agenda for Action: A Report to the Secretary of State for Social Services*, London: HMSO.

Hallam, A., Schneider, J. (1999) Sheltered work schemes for people with mental health problems: Service use and costs. *Journal of Mental Health*, **8** 163–178.

Health Education Authority (1998) *Community action for mental health.* London: Health Education Authority.

Hean, S., Cowley, S., Maben, J., Forbes, A., Griffiths, P. (Research paper in progress, Florence Nightingale School of Nursing and Midwifery, King's College London). *Social Capital: A Concept Analysis.*

Higgins, G., Gianniba, P. (1999) *The Social Firms Directory.* Surrey: Netherne Printing Services and Social Firms UK.

Holmes-Eber, P., Riger, S. (1990) Hospitalisation and the composition of patients' social networks. *Schizophrenia Bulletin*, **16** (1) 157.

Home Office (1999) *Giving Time, Getting Involved: A strategy report by the working group on the active community.* London: Home Office Communication Directorate.

Home Office and Department of Health (1999) *Managing dangerous people with severe personality disorder: Proposals for policy development.* London: Department of Health.

Hughes, A., Walden, S. (1999) Befriending: a note of caution. *British Journal of Learning Disabilities*, **27** (3) 88–92.

Hull, J.T., Thompson, J.C. (1981). Factors which contribute to normalisation in residential facilities for the mentally ill. *Community Mental Health Journal*, **17** 107–113.

Huxley, P., Thornicroft, G. (2000) *Social inclusion and mental health.* London: Health Services Research Department, Institute of Psychiatry.

Janicki, M.P., Ansello, E.F. (eds) (2000) *Community Supports for Aging Adults with Lifelong Disabilities.* Baltimore: Paul H Brookes Publishing.

Jones, J. (1999) *Private Troubles and Public Issues. A Community Development Approach to Health.* Edinburgh: Community Learning Scotland.

Jones, N., Kent, J. (1997) *A Housing and Community Care Strategy for Leeds.* Leeds Joint Consultative Committee.

Kawachi, I., Kennedy, B. *et al.*, (1997) Social Capital, Income Inequality and Mortality. *American Journal of Public Health*, **87** 491–498.

Kawachi, I., Kennedy, B. P., Glass, R. (1999). Social Capital and Self-Rated Health: A Contextual Analysis. *American Journal of Public Health*, **89** 1187–1193.

Kennedy, H. (1997) *Learning Works. Report of the Committee on Widening Participation.* Coventry: Further Education Funding Council.

 © THE SAINSBURY CENTRE FOR MENTAL HEALTH, 2002

Kilpatrick, S. (2000) *How social capital facilitates learning outcomes for small family businesses.* http://www.crla.utas.edu.au/discussion/d2–2000.shtml.

King, N., Harker, M. (2000) *Making Housing Choices.* Brighton: Pavilion Publishing.

Kinsella, P. (1995) *Supported Living – a new paradigm.* Manchester: National Development Team.

Knapp, M., Cambridge, P., Thomason, C., Beecham, J., Allen, C., Darton, R. (1992). *Care in the Community: Challenge and Demonstration.* Aldershot: Ashgate.

Krishna, A., Shrader, E. (1999). *Social Capital Assessment Tool.* http://www.worldbank.org/.

Labonte, R. (1998) *A Community Development Approach to Health Promotion.* Edinburgh: Health Education Board for Scotland.

Leff, J. (1995). Long stay patients seven years after discharge from hospital: outcome. *Tenth Annual Conference of the Team for the Assessment of Psychiatric Services Summary of Proceedings.* London: TAPS.

Leff, J. (1997) (ed) *Care in the Community – Illusion or Reality?* Great Britain: John Wiley & Sons.

Link, B.G., Phelan, J.C. (2001) On the nature and consequences of stigma. *Annual Review of Sociology,* **27** 363–385.

Linszen, D., Birchwood, M. (2000) The Early Phase of Psychosis & Schizophrenia. In Birchwood, M., Fowler, D., Jackson, G. (eds) (2000) *Early Intervention in Psychosis: A Guide to Concepts, Evidence and Interventions.* Chichester: Wiley.

MacDonald–Wilson, K., Whitman, A. (1995) Encouraging disclosure of psychiatric disability: mental health consumer and service provider perspectives on what employers can do. *American Rehabilitation.* Spring 1995, 15–19.

Malpas, G., Weekes, J. (2001) *An Investigation into Drop-ins.* London: Mental Health Foundation.

Marmot, M., Wilkinson, R. (eds) (1999) *The Social Determinants of Health.* Oxford: Oxford University Press.

McGorry, P. (2000) *The Concept of Early Intervention.* In Birchwood, M., Fowler, D., Jackson, G. (eds). *Early Intervention in Psychosis: A Guide to Concepts, Evidence and Interventions,* 6–8. Chichester: Wiley.

Mental Health Foundation (2000a) *In Good Faith.* London: Mental Health Foundation Strategies for Living Project.

Mental Health Foundation (2000b) *Pull yourself together: a survey of stigma and discrimination faced by people who experience mental distress.* London: The Mental Health Foundation.

mentality/The Sainsbury Centre for Mental Health. (2001) *An Executive Briefing on mental health promotion: Implementing Standard One of the National Service Framework.* www.scmh.org.uk.

Mind (2001) *Environmentally Friendly? Patients' views of conditions on psychiatric wards.* London: Mind Publications.

Morgan, W. P. (1997) *Physical Activity and Mental Health.* London: Taylor and Francis.

Muijen, M. (1997) Scare in the Community: Britain in Moral Panic. In Heller, T. *et al.*, (1997) *Mental Health Matters – A Reader,* Chapter 17. Great Britain: Macmillan Press Ltd.

Murray, C. (1990) *The Emerging British Underclass.* London: Institute of Economic Affairs.

Narayan, D. (1998) *Global Social Capital Survey, Republic of Uganda.* http://www.worldbank.org/poverty/scapital/library/narayan2.htm.

 © THE SAINSBURY CENTRE FOR MENTAL HEALTH, 2002

LIBRARY
CHARLES FREARS CAMPUS
DE MONTFORT UNIVERSITY

National Schizophrenia Fellowship has developed a training package for the police. Contact: NSF, 30 Tabernacle St, London EC2A 4DD. Tel 0207 330 9100. http://www.nsf.org.uk.

Nelson, G., Hall, G.B., Squire, D., Walsh–Bowers, R.T. (1992) Social network transactions of psychiatric patients. *Social Science and Medicine*, **34** (4) 433–455.

Newton, C., Wilson, D. (1999) *Circles of Friends*. Dunstable: Folens.

Newton, J., Olson, D., Horner, R. (1995) Factors contributing to the stability of social relationships between individuals with mental retardation and other community members. *Mental Retardation*, **33** 383–393.

Nicholls, V. (2001) *Doing Research Ourselves*. London: Mental Health Foundation.

O'Brien, J. (1987). *A guide to lifestyle planning*. In Wilcox, B., Bellamy, G.T. (eds). *A Comprehensive Guide to the Activities Catalogue. An Alternative Curriculum for Youth and Adults with Severe Disabilities*, 177–185. Baltimore: Paul H Brookes.

O'Brien, J., Lyle O'Brien, C. (2000) *The origins of person-centred planning: a community of practice perspective.* Georgia: USA: Responsive Systems Associates, Inc.

O'Brien, J., Lyle O'Brien, C. (eds). (1999) *A little book about person-centred planning.* Toronto: Inclusion Press.

O'Bryan, A., Simons, K., Beyer, S., Grove, B. (2000) *A Framework for Supported Employment.* York: Joseph Rowntree Foundation/YPS.

Ottenbacher, K.J., Cusick, A. (1993) Discriminative versus evaluative assessment: Some observations on goal attainment scaling. *The American Journal of Occupational Therapy*, **47** 349–354.

Paton, C. (1990) *The Prime Minister's Review of the National Health Service and the 1989 White Paper – Working For Patients.* Social Policy Review.

Peck, E. (2000) Modernising mental health services in a post-modern world, *Journal of Mental Health* (Editorial) **9** (4) 347–350.

Penn, D., Guyan, K., Daily, T. *et al.*, (1994) Dispelling the stigma of schizophrenia: what sort of information is best? *Schizophrenia Bulletin*, **20** (3) 567–574.

Perkins, R., Repper, J. (1996) *Working Alongside People with Long Term Mental Health Problems.* London: Stanley Thornes.

Perkins, R., Buckfield, R., Choy, D. (1997) Access to employment: A supported employment project to enable mental health service users to obtain jobs within mental health teams, *Journal of Mental Health* **6** 307–318.

Pilgrim, D., Waldron, L. (1998) User Involvement in Mental Health Service Development: How Far Can It Go? *Journal of Mental Health*, **7** (1) 95–104.

Pilgrim, D., Rogers, A. (1999) *A Sociology of Mental Health and Illness* (2nd edition). Milton Keynes: Open University Press.

Portes, A., Sessenbrenner, J. (1993) Embeddedness and Immigration: Notes on the Social Determinants of Economic Action. *American Journal of Sociology*, **98** 1320–1350.

Pozner, A., Ng, M.L., Hammond, J., Shepherd, G. (1996) *Working it Out: Creating Work Opportunities for People with Mental Health Problems.* Brighton: Pavilion Publishing.

Priestley, M. (1997) Whose Research? A personal audit. In Barnes, C., Mercer, G. *Doing Disability Research.* Leeds: The Disability Press.

Putnam, R. D. (1993) *Making Democracy Work: Civic Traditions in Modern Italy.* New Jersey: Princeton University Press.

Read, J. (1996) What do we want from mental health services? In Read, J., Reynolds, J. (Eds). *Speaking Our Minds.* Milton Keynes: Open University Press.

Read, J., Baker, S. (1996) *Not just sticks and stones: a survey of the stigma, taboos and discriminations experienced by people with mental health problems.* London: Mind.

Read, J., Harre, N.(2001) The role of biological and genetic causal beliefs in the stigmatisation of 'mental patients'. *Journal of Mental Health,* **10** (2) 223–235.

Repper, J., Brooker, C. (1996) Attitudes towards community facilities for people with serious mental health problems. *Health and Social Care in the Community,* **4** 290–399.

Repper, J., Sayce, L., Strong, S. (1997) *Tall Stories from the Back Yard. A Survey of Nimby Opposition to Community Mental Health Facilities Experienced by Key Service Providers in England and Wales.* London: Mind.

Richardson, A., Ritchie, J. (1989) *Developing Friendships: Enabling People with Learning Difficulties to Make and Maintain Friends.* London: Policy Studies Institute in association with Social and Community Planning Research.

Ritchie, J., Keegan, J. (1983) *Housing for mentally ill and mentally handicapped people.* London: Department of the Environment.

Robson, C. (1993) *Real World Research: A resource for social scientists and practitioner-researchers.* Oxford: Blackwell Publishers Ltd.

Rose, D. (1996) *Living in the Community.* London: The Sainsbury Centre for Mental Health.

Rose, D. (2001) *Users' Voices.* London: The Sainsbury Centre for Mental Health.

Roulstone, A. (2000) Disability, Dependency and the New Deal for Disabled People. *Disability and Society,* **15** (3) 427–443.

The Sainsbury Centre for Mental Health (1999) *NSF for Mental Health Briefing Paper 8.*

The Sainsbury Centre for Mental Health (2000) *On Your Doorstep. Community Organisations and Mental Health.* London: The Sainsbury Centre for Mental Health.

Sanderson, H., Kennedy, J., Ritchie, P., Goodwin, G. (1997) *People, plans and possibilities: exploring person-centred planning.* Edinburgh: Scottish Human Services Trust.

Sartorius, N. (2001) *Global Programme Against Stigma and Discrimination because of Schizophrenia.* Conference presentation, World Psychiatric Association (WPA) Leipzig: 2001.

Sayce, L. (1998) Stigma, Discrimination and Social Exclusion: What's In A Word? *Journal of Mental Health,* **7** (4) 331–343.

Sayce, L. (2000) *From Psychiatric Patient to Citizen. Overcoming Discrimination and Social Exclusion.* Basingstoke: MacMillan.

Sayce, L., Morris, D. (1999) *Outsiders coming in? Achieving social inclusion for people with mental health problems.* London: Mind publications.

Schneider, J. (1998) Models of specialist employment for people with mental health problems, *Health and Social Care in the Community,* **6** (2) 120–129.

Scottish Development Centre for Mental Health (2001a) *Community mental health and well-being. A discussion of concepts and ideas.* Edinburgh: Research Unit in Health, Behaviour and Change, University of Edinburgh.

Scottish Development Centre for Mental Health (2001b) *Report of a seminar on 'Promoting well-being in individuals and communities.* Dundee: 7th June 2001.

 © THE SAINSBURY CENTRE FOR MENTAL HEALTH, 2002

Scottish Office (1999a) *Towards a Healthier Scotland.* Edinburgh: The Stationery Office.

Scottish Office (1999b) *Social Inclusion Strategy: Opening the door to a better Scotland.* Edinburgh: The Stationery Office.

Scottish Public Mental Health Alliance (forthcoming) *Promoting Mental Health and Well-being in Scotland.* A Discussion Paper.

Secker, J., Membrey, H., Grove, B., Seebohm, P., (2001, forthcoming) *The Support and Workplace Adjustments Required for the Success of Open Employment for Mental Health Service Users.*

Sibbet, D. (1981) *"I see what you mean!" An introduction to group graphics.* San Francisco: Sibbet and Associates.

Smale, G., Tuson, G. (1993) *Empowerment, Assessment, Care Management and the Skilled Worker.* London: HMSO.

Smith, R. (1985) Bitterness, shame, emptiness, waste: An introduction to unemployment and health, 1. *British Medical Journal*, **291** 1024–8.

Snijders, T. A. B. (1999) Prologue to the measurement of social capital. *The Tocqueville Review*, **20** 27–44.

Social Exclusion Unit (1999) *What's it all about?* London: Cabinet Office. www.cabinet-office.gov.uk/seu/index/faqs.hmtl.

Sokolovsky, J., Berger, D., Geiger, J. (1978) Personal networks of ex-mental patients in a Manhattan SRO hotel. *Human Organisation*, **3** (7) 4–15.

Standing Nursing and Midwifery Advisory Group – SNMAG (1999) *Addressing Acute Concerns.* London: Department of Health.

Stevens, A., Bur, A., Young, L. (2000) Partial, Unequal and Conflictual: Problems in Using Participation for Social Inclusion in Europe. *Social Work in Europe*, **6** (2) 2–9.

Sudarsky, J. (1999) *Colombia's Social Capital: The National Measurement with the Barcas* (Survey Tool in Spanish). http://www.worldbank.org/poverty/scapital/library/sudarskysurvey.htm.

Tanzman, B. (1993) An overview of surveys of mental health consumers preferences for housing and support services. *Hospital and Community Psychiatry*, **44** 450–455.

Taylor, P., Gunn. J. (1999) Homicides by people with mental illness: myths and reality. *British Journal of Psychiatry*, **174** 9–14.

Thomas, D., Rose, N. (1986) *Getting to Know You. A Reflection and Review of an Individualised Approach to Service Planning.* Manchester: North Manchester Health Authority.

Thomas, D., Holt, V., Illingworth, M., Maddocks, N., Robinson, E. (1990). Designing services with people who are elderly. In Sharkey, S., Barna, S. (eds). *Community Care – People Leaving Long Stay Hospitals.* London: Routledge.

Tomlinson, J. (1996) *Inclusive Learning. Principals and Recommendations: Report of the Learning Difficulties and/or Disabilities Committee.* Coventry: Further Education Funding Council.

Traustadottir, R. (1993) In Amado, A. N. (ed). *Friendships and Community Connections Between People with and without Developmental Disabilities*, 115. Baltimore: Paul H Brookes.

Trivedi, P. (forthcoming May 2002) Racism, social exclusion and mental health – a black user's perspective. In Bhui, K. *Racism and Mental Health: Prejudice and Suffering.* London: Jessica Kingsley.

Turner–Crowson, J. (1997) *Values in Action: First conference proceedings.* London: Bromley Joint Commissioning Department.

 © THE SAINSBURY CENTRE FOR MENTAL HEALTH, 2002

United Nations Special Rapporteur on Disability, Dr Bengt Lindqvist (2001). Speech to a World Health Organisation meeting on *Mental Health and Human Rights.* Geneva: April 2001.

Veiel, H., Baumann, U. (1992) The Many Meanings of Social Support. In Veiel, H., Baumann, U. (eds) *The Meaning and Measurement of Social Support.* Hemisphere Publishing Corporation.

Vernon, A. (1997) Reflexivity: the dilemmas of researching from the inside. In Barnes and Mercer (eds) *Doing Disability Research.* Leeds: The Disability Press.

Wahl, O. (1995) *Media Madness. Public Images of Mental illness.* New Jersey: Rutgers University Press.

Walker, A., Walker, C. (1998) Normalisation and 'normal' ageing: the social construction of dependency among older people with learning difficulties. *Disability and Society,* **13** (1) 125–142.

Warner, R. (1985) *Recovery from schizophrenia: psychiatry and political economy.* London: Routledge and Kegan Paul.

Warner, R. (2000) *The Environment of Schizophrenia. Innovations in Practice, Policy and Communications.* London: Brunner–Routledge.

Watson, L., Tarpey, M. (1998) *Pick and Mix: Developing flexible housing choices in community care.* London: Chartered Institute of Housing.

Webb, D. (2001) *An Investigation into Massage.* London: Mental Health Foundation.

Wehman, P., Revell, W., Kregel, J. (1998) Supported employment; a decade of rapid growth and impact. *American Rehabilitation,* **24** 31–43.

Wertheimer, A. (1997) *Images of Possibility: Creating learning opportunities for adults with mental health difficulties.* Leicester: National Institute for Adult Continuing Education.

Whitaker, P., Barratt, P., Joy, H., Potter, M., Thomas, G. (1998) Children with autism and peer group support: Using circles of friends. *British Journal of Special Education,* **25** (2) 60–65.

Wilmott, P., Thomas, D. (1984) *Community in Social Policy.* London: Policy Studies Institute.

Wolfensberger, W., Glenn, L. (1975) *Program Analysis of Service Systems.* Toronto: National Institute of Mental Retardation.

Wolff, G., Pathare, S., Craig, T., Leff, J. (1996) Community attitudes to mental illness. *British Journal of Psychiatry,* **168** 183–190.

 © THE SAINSBURY CENTRE FOR MENTAL HEALTH, 2002